IN STITCHES

The Diary of a Student Doctor

For my wife, Joan. The best.

IN STITCHES

The Diary of a Student Doctor

Dr John Fleetwood

THE O'BRIEN PRESS
DUBLIN

First published 1994 by The O'Brien Press Ltd.,
20 Victoria Road, Rathgar, Dublin 6, Ireland

British Library Cataloguing-in-publication Data
Fleetwood, John
In Stitches
The Making of an Irish GP
I. Title
610.207

ISBN 0-86278-383-6

10 9 8 7 6 5 4 3 2 1

Typesetting, design and layout: The O'Brien Press Ltd.
Cover illustration: Valerie Byrne
Cover separations: Lithoset, Dublin
Printed in Great Britain by
Cox & Wyman Ltd, Reading, Berkshire

Contents

Preface

A definition of a doctor: an ordinary person thrust into an extraordinary job. This really says it all. Doctors have no claim to special powers or insights. After many years of learning we are given extraordinary responsibilities. We can diagnose problems and treat diseases, but learning about the patient as a person takes years. My father felt he was still on a 'learning curve' after a lifetime in medicine.

I hope this book gives the reader some insight into what medicine is about. When we make mistakes, all we can say is *mea culpa*, and do the best we can. We are ordinary people in an extraordinary job, after all.

Dr John Fleetwood
May 1994

Acknowledgements

This book is about my journey through medical school and training as a junior hospital doctor. Some people deserve my special thanks, especially those who put up with me and taught me. My parents, who started the whole thing off all those years ago, my brother Conor, and my sisters Caroline and Mary, both nurses, who never had any trouble telling me exactly what nurses thought of medical students. To Alison Barnes, our long-suffering secretary, who typed the manuscript and transferred the whole thing onto a floppy disc, whatever that is. And to Frances, my editor in the O'Brien Press, who made me think about things that I would not have thought of, for example, what exactly is a craniotomy?

And finally, to the doctors, both junior and senior, and to the nursing staff and sisters in the wards where I worked, a heart-felt thank you.

Chapter 1

Pre-Med — 1969

'Tony! This boy hasn't got his testicles on the table.'

I looked at the lecturer for a good ten seconds with the smile frozen on my face, wonderful anatomical images flashing by me, as they must have done for the rest of the Pre-Med Zoology class.

Who hadn't got his testicles on the table?

Tony, the long suffering lab attendant, sighed, produced a set of slides from what appeared to be thin air and slapped the relevant ones down in front of the offending student.

'Remember, when examining your testicles, show them to your partner,' instructed the lecturer.

My partner, a very demure girl from the country, blushed like a traffic light and coughed ever so politely. 'She is talking about the *slide*, isn't she?'

It was a few weeks into our Pre-Med year, and if this was anything to go by my life was going to change more than I could have imagined.

University was a very different world from my boarding school in Cashel, County Tipperary. After repeating Sixth Year, I had finally left school. I wanted to join Aer Lingus, but they were not accepting pilots at the time, or so they told me.

If Aer Lingus would not accept me, I thought, at least I

could keep up the family tradition of 'having someone in medicine'. And with my father a GP with a large practice in Dublin, and my mother and both my sisters nurses, this was some tradition. So off I went to university to become a doctor.

Getting into University College Dublin (UCD) was much easier in those days. All you needed was two honours – I had three, I had worked one too hard – and a cheque for fees from the Dad. I was lucky; I was in a very comfortable position. I came from a professional middle-class family with very tolerant parents. I was what you might call a typical sixties teenager, not quite a hippy but leaning in that direction. I had no responsibilities whatsoever except those to myself – and of course the responsibility of getting my mother's car home in one piece after a night on the town.

❖   ❖   ❖   ❖

Between registration and the start of Pre-Med I had decided to look for work. I'd wangled a job as a kitchen boy in a rather old-fashioned psychiatric hospital, no longer in operation. I washed about two thousand pieces of tableware per sitting, and built up an everlasting hatred for washing-up. When I begged to be assigned to another part of the hospital, the manager said 'No'. I was replacing the main 'washer-upper' who had suffered a nervous breakdown and been diagnosed as a paranoid schizophrenic. It was pure luck, I was told, that he happened to be working in a psychiatric hospital at the time.

It was in that hospital that one of the chefs pointed to the eggs in the huge frying pans and told me they were 'made by the girls'. I became a little suspicious when he pointed to little bits and pieces of fat in the pan and asked: 'Do you think that this is the sperm?'

My knowledge of hen biology was not up to the required standard of the kitchen, I decided, and I backed away towards the door looking frantically for something with which to defend myself. But the wooden spoon I snatched up was no match for the enormous kitchen knife the chef had tucked away in his belt. I like to think that I left that job shortly afterwards of my own volition!

For the remaining six weeks before term began I became a porter/gofer/'consultant' (after all I was going to Med School) in a large geriatric home. I opted for night duty as the pay was considerably better than for day duty and worked from 8pm to 8am five days a week. My colleagues in 'portership' were in a constant state of altered consciousness brought on by inhaling illegal substances. They also smoked about twenty cigarettes per shift and, whether feeding patients, washing up, or eating food, had one constantly in their mouths. Not only that but they also made sure the patients had a good supply of tobacco. Still, they weren't always sure what exactly happened to it. One night, as I sat with another porter at the end of a long corridor, we saw, with some interest, a patient stumbling towards us wearing nothing but a tie. He was leaving a little trail behind him. We found that it was made up of a wad of tobacco which was poking out of his bum. 'So! That's where he has been shoving all his fags!' said my colleague. He took hold of the old gent's tie and led him back to his room.

The porters also occasionally actually gave out the tablets and made tentative diagnoses, always deferring to the senior porter who was so long at the job that he gave suppositories without using a glove. He was regarded with some awe. I like to believe that it was not my fault that the prescribed medications would sometimes get mixed up. One of the nursing staff was fond of the booze and on the odd occasion she would be more comatose than her charges. We porters, therefore, had to figure out for ourselves which medication was intended for which patient.

Six weeks in this home prepared me for the shock of dealing with 'body fluids'. Every morning at six o'clock when we washed and changed our patients, there would be bowel movements everywhere. Door, sink, floor, everything would be covered. All kinds of body fluids were hurled around. Some of the patients even appeared to use them for finger painting. At first I felt a bit sick, but like all things in medicine you do get used to it. It was a relief to leave my summer jobs behind and actually begin Pre-Med.

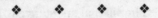

It was the late sixties in UCD and the 'Lefties' were much in evidence. They used to congregate in the café of the Science Block. Whenever we went for a cup of coffee between lectures they were there and they got up everybody's nose. One of us med students targeted these people without mercy. He would stand near those who were selling the *Daily Worker* and hand out *Time* and *Newsweek*. One day he decided to take the law into his own hands. He presented himself at one of their tables.

'I would like to join the Connolly Youth Movement,' he said deadpan.

'Fan-bloody-tastic, Comrade. Let me show you some literature on our movement.'

'I have just one question,' he added.

'And what's that, Comrade?'

'When is your dress dance?'

The fight that followed was great entertainment and the only damage done was to the reputation of the Lefties. They realised they were not being taken very seriously and disappeared off to the Arts Block, where any student who joined their cause was instantly renamed an Arsehole Recruited To Socialism or ARTS. But the closest I ever got to left-wing was to chase some of the girls I thought would be more morally lax than the others.

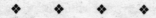

Pre-med covered physics, Chemistry, Zoology, and of all things, Botany. Botany was a hangover from the old days when doctors used plants and herbs to treat their victims. Our Botany lecturer, now dead, was a kindly old priest who hated failing students. This was used to great advantage before exams when one or two girls would go to his rooms, crying and bemoaning the fact that they were overworked, had to get part-time jobs to support themselves and were dreadfully worried about the exam. Within thirty minutes the lecturer would have given them some very strong hints as to what to study for the examinations. Naturally they passed this information on to the rest of the class. That year nobody failed Botany.

But I did fail Physics and I had to repeat the year. To help pass the time I took a job as a part-time ambulance man with a private ambulance service, which had set up an advanced mobile cardiac unit. It was one of the most modern in Europe and set the standard for future mobile cardiac services.

The crews were made up of two firemen doing 'nixers' and other guys who drifted in and out. For the first few weeks I was merely the hanger-on when we went out on an emergency. But I felt a certain thrill, even a little arrogance, when we blasted our way through the traffic. The ambulances had American sirens, not bells, and a few people thought that

UFOs were about to land when they first heard them!

My first cardiac arrest experience was on New Year's Eve with a call to a hotel where a diner had keeled over.

The hotel was at the top of a hill with a fairly long driveway. Unfortunately, the driveway was blocked by cars and we had to charge through a narrow passageway with the stretcher loaded down with the various pieces of machinery and monitors. We ran into the dining-hall expecting a hushed crowd. Not exactly. The music was still blaring, people were dancing and singing and the unfortunate man was tucked away under a long table at which people were still sitting. We had to do something. We dragged the body out to the lobby and put on a show. The people around were expecting us to save lives. Not this one.

After a few minutes' show of cardiac massage and mouth-to-mouth resuscitation, we knew we were on to a loser. We set up the defibrillator. This machine restarts the heart by passing a huge charge of electricity via two paddles into the patient's heart, shocking it back to its normal rhythm. We shocked the body once or twice, put it on the stretcher and wheeled it to the hotel door. The ambulance was about thirty yards down the drive at the bottom of the hill. Somehow the stretcher escaped us. Off it went by itself, neatly rolling between the rows of parked cars. I charged after it, caught it and unfortunately tripped and ended up on the stretcher with the body. Finally, the ambulance put a stop to our macabre journey at the cost of a broken headlight.

After a few months I had enough experience to be allowed out with only the driver. My only knowledge of trauma was from my stint with the Order of Malta when I was about thirteen years old. However well you are trained by the good Order, it does not prepare you for, say, decapitation. That was somewhat rare when you were on duty in the Order of

Malta hut by the seaside putting iodine on cut feet. But the firemen and full-time ambulance men I worked with taught me more about dealing with trauma and immediate care of the injured than all the professors were to do in Med School. I saw the big, tough firemen weep when a child died, banging their fists against the wall in frustration when a doctor made a complete mess of resuscitation.

Dealing with messy cases was part of the job. You slowly got used to it. Even hardened firemen who thought they had seen it all were occasionally caught totally unprepared. There was an accident close to the ambulance station and one night myself and two very experienced firemen were called out. A car had ploughed into a wall and the engine had been pushed back, quite literally, onto the driver's lap, squashing his abdomen. He was still alive when we arrived, mumbling in pain. I stood near the wreck, rooted to the spot. It was hopeless, nothing could be done for the poor man. One of the firemen bent down to give him some type of comfort and looked directly into the driver's eyes. All the man said was 'Help me, help me, please help me,' over and over, softer and softer, until his head tilted forward and he died. The fireman straightened up with tears streaming down his face. 'I couldn't help, I just couldn't help,' he said.

We knocked off early that night and the three of us got blind drunk.

At first I had great difficulty when we got back to the ambulance station after very traumatic accidents. But the firemen were very practical. They would brew up a cup of tea, talk about what had happened and that was that. It was the best counselling I ever got. The very black humour that I thought sick at first was also their way of warding off the awful things they dealt with every day.

One of the firemen, Paddy, was a very experienced crew

member and we worked together on many occasions in the ambulance. He had the reputation of getting the 'odd ones', a bit of a jinx if you like. I always felt a tinge of excitement on call with him. With Paddy it was bound to be something different.

We were sent one morning to collect a body. When we arrived at the house, the door was opened by a little old man. He was as daft as a pole. He looked at our uniforms and decided we were the police.

'What do you want, Officer?' he asked.

'We've come to collect the body.'

'What body?' he said, suspiciously.

'The body that's dead,' said my partner Paddy.

'What body is dead?' his eyes narrowed.

I was beginning to feel exasperated. 'The body, the bloody dead body somewhere in this kip.'

Paddy whimpered and called up the controller on the two-way radio for more details.

He returned armed with the corpse's name and apartment number.

'Sir, we have to collect a body from the downstairs flat, Flat 2,' he said, and gave the old man the name of the lady who had died.

'She's gone to Australia to visit her son. He has a Rolls Royce. He is going to convert it into flats,' was the reply.

For a few moments we were at a loss for words.

'May we come in and have a look?' I asked eventually.

'Why?'

'If there is a body in Flat 2, we'd like to remove it. Otherwise it might get a bit smelly,' Paddy said. The old man reluctantly opened the door a few inches and we squeezed in. The smell hit us like a brick.

'Oh, no,' croaked Paddy. 'It's rotten already.'

We opened the door to Flat 2, not daring to breathe. We could taste the smell. It was everywhere. It crawled all over us. Lying in a bed in the corner of the room was a very dead old lady. Nothing had been touched. We reckoned that the police had taken a very quick look at the room, decided against foul play and beaten a hasty retreat. We ran back out to the ambulance to get the trolley, and take a few deep breaths.

We put the stretcher down beside the bed, lowered it to the ground and pulled back the covers. In the bed was a tiny female body, nearly black and stiff as a board. She looked like she weighed about four stone. I took her by the ankles and Paddy put his hands under her head. Unfortunately, halfway between the bed and the trolley she bent in the middle. This movement acted like a bellows and ejected the remaining contents of her bowel in a little jet from her rectum. I was covered with stuff that looked like it came from a swamp. I screamed and let her drop. This had the same effect on her top half where, unfortunately, her face was turned towards Paddy.

Paddy had always said that he had seen it all. He hadn't. We ran from the room, wrestling with each other to get out of the door first, and collapsed in the hall. Paddy vomited onto the carpet and I ripped off my shoes, socks and trousers and threw them out the door onto the street.

The old fella was now somewhere in a mass of smoke, puffing frantically on a pipe.

He poked his finger at Paddy. 'You'll have to clean that up, Sergeant,' he said.

Paddy looked at him with the face of one who had tasted hell and told him in no uncertain terms what he was going to do and where he was going to shove his pipe, tobacco and all.

The mayhem had attracted passers-by who gathered at the front door, mouths open, gawking at the scene – two uniformed men, one kneeling on the floor over a pile of evil-smelling material, threatening a little old man enveloped in pipesmoke, the other, with no trousers on, dancing an Irish jig, and shouting, 'Oh shit! Oh shit! Shit!' My trousers lay on the step just outside the front door. A dog came up to them, smelled them, cocked his leg and peed on them.

When we arrived at the morgue, nobody mentioned that I had no trousers on, that Paddy looked as if his hair was standing on end, or that the ambulance smelt like a sewer. That night, however, I went out with a girl on our first-and-final date. I subsequently found out that she did not like me because I 'smelt funny'.

Paddy became a good friend and remained so after I left the services and became a doctor. Some years later the doorbell rang and there stood Paddy with his wife. He looked awful. He looked as if he was in pain.

'John, I've got a terrible headache,' he whispered.

The next day a scan showed a tumour in his brain. Other tests showed the lung cancer that had spawned the brain tumour. Paddy died a few months later. Not only had I lost a patient, I had lost a good friend.

❖   ❖   ❖   ❖

I passed my pre-med repeats that summer. The next day I saved my first life.

I arrived at work in the morning and sat down for a cup of coffee. Immediately, the alarm bells shattered the early morning fog that was slowly lifting from my brain. These bells, I suspect, were designed to sound like huge alarm clocks. Away we went on a cardiac to the northside of the city, a journey of about twenty miles. We stopped outside a large country house where we were met by a young woman and her family. In the bedroom her husband was very pale and sweating. We put him in the ambulance and raced off to the hospital. He was hooked up to the monitors and kept lapsing in and out of consciousness. Initially the heartbeat on the monitor had a smooth rhythm but as we got closer to the hospital it started to show irregular beats. I glanced away from the monitor for a moment and when I looked back it showed the wavy line of ventricular fibrillation, a condition where the heart loses its ability to pump blood. His heart had stopped!

I yelled: 'Arrest,' and the driver slammed on the brakes and pulled into the side of the road. I thumped the patient's chest very hard with my fist, then pumped it with both hands, trying to force blood up to his brain. After about four minutes without oxygen the brain begins to die and, even if revived, a victim can suffer brain damage. The driver fired up the defibrillator and placed both paddles on the man's chest and fired the electrical charge. The man leapt off the stretcher just like they do in the movies. I looked back at the monitor. A gentle beep, beep cut across the screen. We had restarted his heart! A great big smile appeared on our faces. We made sure he was breathing by himself and raced off to the hospital. Within ten minutes of his cardiac arrest he was in the coronary care unit.

I saw him recently in my surgery for a check-up. His ECG showed the legacy of his heart attack more than twenty years ago. But he is now a grandfather and his children and grandchildren are my patients.

Chapter 2

First Med

First Med began that October. At last I was into real medicine. Well, not exactly *real* medicine. Before we students were allowed to touch a patient we had to learn how their bodies worked. Our major subjects were Physiology, Anatomy and Biochemistry, with minor subjects like Ethics thrown in for good measure. The Ethics lectures were held in the afternoons which gave us a super excuse to have a nap.

My first sight of the anatomy lab gave me shivers all over. A few of us stood nervously at the door. There were twelve dead bodies on benches. One had a lighted cigarette in his mouth. We never found out who put it there.

The senior lecturer appeared through another door at the end of the lab.

'Come in! Come in, they won't bite!' he called heartily and ushered us to our respective bodies. There was one body for each group of eight students, more than enough. We got a lecture on respecting the bodies and the generosity of the patients and their families in contributing their bodies to science. There was to be no messing with the bodies, our lecturer warned.

A few years previously, as the story went, a body had been 'borrowed' from one of the medical schools and ended up in a very posh Dublin hotel. It was only when the *maître d'* tried to extract the price of dinner for four that he noticed his diner was dead.

There was also the story of the skeleton two medical students had taken, wrapped up in clothes, hat and scarf and put on the back seat of their car. They picked up a charming American exchange student who was hitch-hiking. She left the car screaming hysterically when the skeleton's head fell onto her lap.

The lecturer explained that he wanted us to open the abdomen. He demonstrated on one of the bodies. It looked easy enough. But when we stood around the body nobody wanted to make the first move. I picked up the scalpel. My first cut into the abdomen brought my stomach into my mouth. I cut through the skin and into the fat and suddenly an intestine popped out. Not much, but enough to make us cry, 'Oh shit, shit!'

We backed away, half expecting the body to sit up.

'Good, good,' said the lecturer. 'Incise the whole abdominal wall and expose the omentum and mesentery as demonstrated.' He walked off.

'The *what?*' I asked. 'What is the omentum and the pheasantry?'

'I thought he said a monastery,' said another.

We leaned over the body, peering at the little bit of intestine that beckoned us to explore. With an intake of breath, one of the other students enlarged the opening, cutting from the bottom of the breast down to the pubic bone. We hadn't a clue what we were looking for.

In the first months we always wore gloves but gradually we became used to the bodies. By the end of the Anatomy year, gloves were a thing of the past. A brief wash was sufficient to remove the bits and pieces on our hands and lurking under our fingernails.

My father used to tell me story of an anatomy lecturer many

years ago when he was a student. This man liked to smoke a pipe during demonstrations on the various parts of the body. What upset the students was that he would use his pipe stem to move the organs around. He would then wipe the stem on his coat and pop it back in his mouth. He was a man I would love to have met.

❖   ❖   ❖   ❖

I was sitting on the bus home one sunny evening when the conductor came round for the fare. I grabbed a handful of change from my jacket pocket. But when I tried to pick out the exact fare, there in the palm of my hand was an eyeball staring up at me. Someone must have slipped it into my jacket pocket during the Anatomy practical.

The bus conductor bent close. 'What the hell is that?'

'A marble,' I stammered. 'A plastic marble.'

'Looks like an eyeball to me.'

'Nah, a marble. Who'd leave an eyeball in their pocket?'

'I wouldn't know, would I?' he said and looked pointedly at my *Grey's Anatomy*, the bible of Anatomy students. 'You wouldn't be the first bloody medical student I've picked up at that stop.'

He took my money and went on collecting other fares. I sat back in my seat, my thoughts somewhat jumbled. What did he mean, not the first medical student? Had he come across others producing kidneys, spleens, maybe a whole liver out of their pockets? I never got to ask him.

❖   ❖   ❖   ❖

Anatomy was meant to teach us students about the organs .of the body; Physiology showed us how those organs worked.

Lectures made up a sizeable portion of our year. We also had tutorials and practicals. Usually these were straightforward but occasionally we actually became the guinea pigs.

At one practical we compared the amount of urine produced after a student took a pint of water with glucose, or a pint of water with salt, or an ordinary pint of water, or a pint of water after an injection of ADH, a hormone that stops the production of urine. I volunteered for the ADH injection, and we all drank the water. The practical lasted two hours and during that time all the class passed urine except me. I had been invited to a party in the Isle of Man that night. That afternoon I went to the airport. I still hadn't taken a piddle. On the plane I met a very nice bloke, full of chat. The flight lasted only forty minutes but we managed to have three gin and tonics each. Alcohol hits my head like a pile driver and when I met my host I was far from sober. And I still had not passed water.

Off we went to a pub in Douglas where we lowered numerous pints and chatted up the talent. I managed to corner one of the local beauties and proceeded to use the best chat-up lines I could conjure up. Five pints later, I thought that we were getting along famously, but suddenly, the effect of that morning's injection wore off and my bladder was out to exact revenge. I tried to explain to the beauty about the ADH, but the physiology of urine production was not something she wanted to chat about. I think she thought I was a little odd. After my tenth visit to the toilets she abandoned me, leaving me hopping from foot to foot like a little boy holding his bladder. Other guests asked my host if I had a prostate problem – a little unusual in someone of my age. I still harbour the suspicion that I got a shot of ADH a mite stronger than intended.

Another practical dealt with the effect of hyperventilating

with pure oxygen on holding one's breath. One of the students did over five minutes. He refused to breathe even though he had collapsed on the floor and was twitching a little. He refused until the lecturer, who was white with fright, actually shook him by the shoulders and pleaded with him to inhale. He finally did, much to the disappointment of the students who were chanting, 'Six minutes, six minutes, easy, easy.' There were other practicals in which we became guinea pigs but none as exciting as this. It was not every day that the Physiology class had an opportunity to watch a fellow student nearly kill himself through willpower alone.

At the end of First Med I scraped through the exams. Now I had a long summer in front of me. I had learnt about many things during that first year – the way the body works, how to approach exams and where the nurses' home in St Vincent's was going to be built!

❖   ❖   ❖   ❖

One of my distant relatives was a nurse in a London hospital. She arranged for me to become a night porter for the summer at the incredible salary of £70 a week. I arrived by train in London in July, phoned a friend and set off for his flat in one of the shabbier parts of town. The door was opened, not by my friend, but by a fellow whose hair appeared to be on fire. He was wearing John Lennon-type sunglasses and was smoking a 'joint'.

'Wha!' he said. 'Wha' do you want?'

I think he was English and human but the point could be argued.

'I'm looking for Liam,' I said. The smell of the smoke was getting up my nose. 'Liam O'Connor.'

'Oh,' he beamed. 'You mean the one who works?'

I nodded. Little did Liam's employers know who his flatmates were. Liam's employers were a very large chemical company whose chemicals were a little more legal than those his flatmates were smoking and shoving up their noses. Liam's flatmates were, for want of a better word, drug pushers for the rock groups and bands in and around London. We did not get on at all. The flat had three bedrooms, one tiny bathroom and filthy kitchen where only toast was ever made. I stayed there for two weeks, sharing a bed with a bloke who went out during the day so I could sleep and slept in the bed at night when I went to work. Liam never did tell me how he met up with these people. Then I moved into a flat with three total strangers, two nurses and an American who was a stocks and shares analyst. This was my first time away from home. I had every intention of meeting as many girls as possible, but the best laid plans ... I worked as many shifts as I could and had little time left to explore the nurses' home.

Tony was one of my fellow porters and he had a decidedly morbid sense of humour. When we were called to collect a body in one of the wards one night Tony went to the nurses' station and said, 'Bring out your dead! Bring out your dead.' He upset a few of the junior surgeons in the surgical wards when, if a patient had died, Tony said he had come to remove 'the mistakes'. The other porters in the hospital were the usual bunch of weirdos and misfits who usually ended up on night duty. During my travels through medical school and my various holiday jobs, I noticed that those who did night duty tended to be one short of a dozen – a fact not lost on my parents.

I occasionally worked as a casualty porter. I thought that my time with the ambulance service would have prepared me for what I saw in the emergency room but this was not the case. One night, a young girl was brought in with a branch of a tree literally sticking through her right eye. She died very soon afterwards. I stood at the end of her stretcher and looked at the body when all the resuscitation equipment had been moved away. Someone had forgotten to take off the heart monitor leads and the straight line across the monitor hypnotised me.

A nurse brushed by me and switched off the monitor. She turned towards me, tears streaming down her face. 'So young, so young,' was all she said.

I left the cubicle to go outside for a breath of fresh air. The surgical registrar who had tried to resuscitate the girl was also crying. 'Sometimes I hate this bloody job,' he said. In the years to come I would know exactly what he meant.

❖　　❖　　❖　　❖

Shortly after I arrived back in Dublin I heard that the cardiology department in one of the hospitals was looking for a research student for the remaining few weeks of the summer holidays. Why not? I thought to myself. I introduced myself to the research registrar and told him I was available for the job if it was still open. It was. I had the job on one condition.

'Have you taken blood before?' he asked

I hadn't, ever. The only veins I had ever attacked were those in dead bodies in the Anatomy classes. 'Many times,' I stammered.

'Can you do blood pressure?'

Well, I had, in theory. I nodded. 'A few times but not very often.'

'Come to the lipid clinic tomorrow and you can start.'

The lipid clinic was where patients' cholesterol and other blood fat levels were investigated and treated if necessary. Blood samples had to be taken from each patient. The job was for three weeks and paid £25 in all.

I arrived at the crowded clinic the next morning. The research registrar pointed to the first cubicle and told me to start taking blood samples. I pulled back the curtains of the cubicle and found a huge man sitting on the couch. He was a docker and must have weighed 25 stone. A big, tough, hairy docker. With trembling hands, I opened a syringe and needle packet and put a tourniquet around his massive biceps. For a brief moment I could think of nothing but Soviet air hostesses. He held his arm out and I made my first jab at his bulging vein. It looked like a motorway on a road map. How could I miss? I did, and hit his tendon. I saw his eyes opening in pain but he did not flinch. He took a deep breath and looked down at the offending weapon standing into his arm.

'New student?' he asked casually.

'Yes,' I mumbled. I withdrew the needle inspecting the syringe for any residue – blood, piece of tendon, skin, anything.

'Ever taken blood before?' he enquired.

I had to tell him the truth, 'No. Never. You're the first.'

'Ok.' He took a deep breath, and said, 'Go ahead.'

He only coughed once when I plunged the needle wildly into his elbow. I was beginning to get hysterical when, wonders of wonders, 'red crude' appeared in the syringe. I filled the tube and withdrew the needle, thrilled and happy. I was squirting the blood into the sample tube when he coughed gently for a second time. I turned around and saw that there was a pool of blood on the floor. I had forgotten to take off the tourniquet.

I undid it and started to wipe up the blood with a towel. I had to take his blood pressure too so I wrapped the cuff of the blood pressure apparatus around his other arm. I puffed up the cuff and put my stethoscope to his elbow. I had a vague idea what to listen for.

I heard nothing.

The head of the stethoscope was practically surrounded by fat. I looked directly into his eyes. He must have seen the sweat breaking out on my forehead. I still had not deflated the cuff and his arm was going blue.

'Doc,' he said, 'the last time my blood pressure was done was ten days ago. It was 180/100 then and I'm sure it is going to be the same today. Why don't you take that yoke off my arm before it turns black and let's pretend nothing has changed. OK?'

Could I refuse a guy who probably ate puppies for his supper? I removed the cuff sheepishly, whispered my thanks and left the cubicle.

The registrar came up to me. 'Any problems?'

'No, none at all. Easy as pie.'

A little old lady was waiting in the next cubicle. Compared to the docker she was a piece of cake. Not only did I get the blood on my first try but I also read her blood pressure. My first blood. I had come through my baptism of fire. I went through the rest of the patients like a dose of salts, whipping blood out of them with impunity. I tested about twenty-five people that day. I was thrilled and happy. The registrar came to me at the end of the day and looked at the neat rows of sample tubes.

'Lovely, well done. Who does this one belong to?'

'Sorry?' I said.

'You forgot to label the tubes, idiot!' he roared.

I had forgotten to label a number of the blood tubes and the patients would have to be recalled. My punishment was to buy the registrar a few pints in our local, the Merrion Inn.

I finished my three-week stint in the cardiology department, humbler and wiser and prepared for Second Med.

Chapter 3

Second Med

Second Med continued where First Med had left off, with the emphasis on the anatomy and physiology of the neck and head, especially the brain. We were still not allowed to see patients, but a greater variety of diseases was put our way.

One day, well into Second Med, I came across an article in a magazine about a controversy between some famous heart surgeons in the USA. Second Med students had a very long summer vacation and I hadn't decided what to do yet. Most students invaded the shores of the USA and worked at any job – legal or illegal – they could get away with. Medical students did not *have* to work in a hospital but it was a good opportunity to gain experience.

I wrote to both surgeons asking for a job. Weeks passed. At last a letter came from one of the surgeons telling me in a very nice way to get lost. A few days later I got a letter from the other surgeon's administrator which held out much more hope.

Although their student places were now full, wrote the administrator, they were considering a place for a foreign extern or student doctor from overseas with suitable references. He also made it clear that I should have some clinical experience. That created a small problem. A medical student had to have completed Third Med in Ireland to have had any clinical experience. I would be just into Third Med with very little clinical experience. But here was a chance that was too good to miss.

I juggled the amount of time I had been in medical school and felt that four years seemed about right. Now for the references. These had to be very good as there would be great competition for the extern position. What could I do to beat the other candidates?

I managed to acquire references that were to my benefit. These said nothing about clinical experience, but mentioned that I had worked as a research student and that I was interested in cardiology. I sent these off and waited with bated breath. Some weeks later I received a letter from the States. I was in! I was speechless. I was going to be an extern student to one of the world's most famous cardiac surgeons.

In preparation, I asked some of the surgeons in Dublin if I could watch operations so at least I'd have some idea what went on in the operating theatres. Little did I know then that my three months in America would turn out to be one of the most exciting periods of my life, but not in cardiac surgery. I would find myself in neurosurgery.

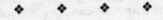

America — The first Trip

I arrived in the USA on a Sunday evening. My quarters were in the residence of the College of Medicine, right next door to the hospital where the famous surgeon worked. I had a bite to eat and went out for a walk, was nearly mugged and returned rapidly to my apartment. Even so, I soon fell into an exhausted and wonderful sleep.

The next morning, fresh and eager, I presented myself to the medical administrator who informed me I was one of only two foreign students accepted out of three hundred and sixteen. Unfortunately, the administrator continued, the surgeon's team had its quota of students at the moment. Would I mind being assigned to the accident and emergency room (casualty) in the general hospital?

I was aware of the emergency rooms (ER) in Dublin, but I had never been a student in one. I was also four thousand miles from home and I could hardly refuse.

The doctor in charge looked me up and down. 'In there,' he said, pointing to a room off the main area. 'Start suturing.' Suturing is a fancy word for stitching, putting people back together again.

'Sorry?' I said incredulously. I had never sutured a person in my life. I had a good idea how stitches were put in, but had yet to actually *do* it.

'I'm told you're a fourth year medical student. Right?' he said.

'Something like that,' I mumbled.

'You take charge of the suture room. There's nobody else. There are no other students in this ER at the moment. For the next week you're the only one. OK?'

I took a deep breath and followed him to the suture room which was already full of patients with various-sized cuts, lacerations and wounds. They all needed to be stitched. What on earth was I going to do?

'You want me to stitch all these people, right now?' I asked.

'Students sew, buddy. OK?'

I was in a dilemma – being a smart arse had got me the job, now it was pay-back time.

'Sure. One small problem. Maybe we suture a different way at home. Could you show me how you do it over here?'

He thought this was a fair question and much to my relief put two sutures into a black fellow's hand. He put the sutures in so fast that all I saw was a blur of motion.

'That's how it's done, Irish.' And off he went.

The patient looked at me, no doubt wondering when I was going to finish the wound in his hand. I put on a pair of gloves and took up the suture forceps. With a deep breath, I plunged the needle in. Luckily the wound had been anaesthetised so the patient did not scream when I put the needle through a tendon. There were more than twenty people, all black, all waiting for me. What the hell, I thought. Just do it.

An hour later the doctor came back to check up. I think he was a little puzzled by some of the scars, the first few looked like a demented plastic surgeon had been at work. However, with each patient I improved and, after the first twenty, I felt I could attempt any skin wound that presented itself.

At the front of the ER were the shock rooms where very seriously injured people were worked on, people who were in shock.

Outside these rooms the corridors were pockmarked with bullet holes where people had fired their guns in anger. When I was shown around the accident and emergency rooms, these bullets holes were pointed out with honour and pride. This was a tough area.

My first night on duty I stood open-mouthed at the trauma cases that were presented in the shock rooms. Here, a patient's wounds were assessed and they were then despatched to the operating room or wherever necessary. The first case was an abdominal knife wound and was removed promptly to the operating room (ORC). The second case was a huge black guy with a shotgun wound to the chest. I asked if I could watch the operation.

'Watch? Hell, kid, you can assist,' said the chief chest cutter.

'I beg your pardon?' I said. The United States was not turning out as I had imagined. Assisting at emergency chest surgery was not on my agenda.

'Listen, kid, this is an emergency hospital. We all work. Where are you from anyway? England?' The ultimate insult!

'I'm Irish. Very little experience in chest surgery.' No experience, I wanted to shout, in any type of surgery, chest or whatever.

'So you'll learn, kid.' I wanted to run away. Instead I watched him as he scrubbed his hands. I watched every move he made as we put on our scrub suits.

The gunshot victim was wheeled down and the surgeon opened his chest. Instinctively, I swabbed at the blood, fascinated at the operation going on under my eyes. It was the first time I had ever seen a beating heart. Little shotgun pellets littered the left ventricle wall.

The surgeon handed me a pair of forceps. 'Go on, try and get one,' he said.

I tried to catch the pellets in the great big beating heart. The surgeon did much better. The pile of x-rays had shown about twenty pellets embedded in a muscle but after an hour or so we had only found sixteen, fourteen for him against two for me. The surgeon decided that if the big guy could survive a shotgun blast to the chest, he could get along with three or four 'rinky-dinky little pellets stuck in his ticker'. He closed the chest, did what was necessary and finished up. I closed the skin.

The operation ended with no fuss, no dramatics. I had seen my first operation – I had *assisted* at my first operation and nobody seemed to care. And why should they? This trauma hospital was one of the busiest trauma hospitals in the world. Gunshot wounds were routine. Back home a gunshot wound would be a major talking point in the coffee shop.

I went back to the ER where the suture room was already full again. The shock rooms were also busy. A sixteen-year-old boy was brought in with a gunshot wound to his spine. He was paralysed and would be for the rest of his life. A young child with some form of bizarre neurological catastrophe was wheeled in, convulsing uncontrollably. By the time he was taken to the paediatric intensive care unit he was, according to the admitting doctor, 'really up the creek'. A young girl was brought in with a knife slash to her face. She looked as if she had been pretty once, not any more.

It was now five in the morning. I had started my surgical extern rotation at eleven the previous morning. I had learned how to suture, had assisted at a heart operation, had watched trauma of all shapes and sizes coming into the shock rooms, all on my very first day – a quiet day according to the staff. Mondays usually were. They said that the weekend of a full moon was another matter altogether and one of these monsters was approaching.

❖   ❖   ❖   ❖

One of the stranger incidents I came across happened a few days later. I was near the shock rooms when a tall black guy came up behind me and tapped me on the shoulder.

'Hey honky, I've been knifed in the belly,' he said. He had no shirt on. I looked at his abdomen but could see nothing. He had his right hand on his right side, casual-like. No blood, nothing to indicate a wound.

'Oh yes,' I said, 'and where in the belly were you knifed?' I think I sniggered a little.

'Here, you white trash!' He took his right hand away. He certainly had been knifed in the belly. His intestines started pouring out. I was dumbstruck.

'Whatcha goin' to do, yo' big muddah?' he shouted. His voice was loud enough to bring desperately needed help. He was dragged into a shock room and put on the table. A significant part of his small intestine had squeezed out of the wound. His trousers and underpants were removed.

'Hey, Irish,' shouted one of the interns, 'bung him up on an IV.' I took hold of his hand put on a tourniquet and slipped in the drip needle. The patient, whom I shall call Norman, got angry. He sprang up from the table with a roar, hitting two doctors in the face as he did so. I fell back into the instrument cabinet. Norman ran out of the room, naked, his guts hanging out. We raced after him and finally cornered him in the holding area. He jumped up on to a stretcher holding on to his intestines as if he was holding a piece of rope. He put his fist through the roof. I stood there amazed. Things like this did not happen at home.

The nurse beside me was very relaxed about the whole affair. 'Norman, you get down from there right now. We want to put your guts back in.'

Norman swung his intestines around like a lasso. One of the older and more experienced doctors nodded towards him. 'It's drugs. Probably amphetamines and cocaine. It makes them think they're invincible. We'll patch him up tonight and he'll discharge himself in about four days. The sutures will still be in. Get one of the local doctors to fix things up for him. He'll be back here in a few weeks. He'll be dead in a year, silly bastard.'

We finally calmed Norman down and brought him to the OR where he was opened up for the second time that night and the wound in his intestine was repaired. I was invited to assist the very strange general surgical resident on duty. The surgeon asked for a small surgical knife and it disappeared into Norman's abdomen. It came back out with a tiny sliver of Norman's liver on the blade. It was put up to my startled eyes.

'Irish, you will never get another chance,' the surgeon said. He appeared to be chewing something.

'Another chance to what?' I hoped he didn't mean what I thought.

'Try the liver,' he whispered.

Whether I did or didn't is a secret that will go with me to my grave.

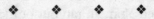

It was a short time after this that I met the man who would teach me more about surgery than anybody else. This second-generation Irish neurosurgeon – Patrick, or Pat – was a bachelor who loved women. He was also financially independent, and was doing neurosurgery because 'Well, gee, it's fun, John!'

His junior colleague, Sean, was also a second-generation Irishman. It seemed ironic to me that I had come all the way to the United States to meet two Irish neurosurgeons.

My first meeting with Pat took place over one of the worst cases I had seen in the shock rooms. I wandered in one day and gasped at the sight before me. The patient had no head. He had the remains of a face but no head. He had put both barrels of a shotgun into his mouth. He had also put a small whiskey glass into his mouth before he used the gun. This guy really wanted to die.

A big, potbellied cop, chewing tobacco, was staring at the remains. He cleared his throat and spat a wad of tobacco juice into the corner. 'This guy's brains are all over his living-room wall,' he said in a heavy American drawl. 'We need a scraper to remove the mess.' I think it was mere curiosity that had brought him to see the wounds.

A neurosurgeon looked up from the head wound. 'Shit!' he said. 'We couldn't even get his damn kidneys.' He looked over at me, 'You the Irish medical student?'

'You can tell?' I stammered.

'Yep. You're the only one that's turned green.'

I could feel the bile in my throat.

'I need an assistant on Monday in surgery.'

'I have no interest in neurosurgery,' I answered.

'Join me. I'll make you interested. Seven in the morning, operating room number 1.' Pat left the shock room. He left me there, wondering what I had got myself into.

I came across Pat quite often that weekend as he inspected the gunshot wounds in patients' heads. I think that the city must have been sold out of the neat little guns called Saturday Night Specials that weekend. Whenever a live patient came in and was conscious I would ask who had shot him or her. The answer was always, 'A friend'. Some very odd friends were to be found in town.

That Sunday night the effects of the full moon came to a head. I was in the suture room when the shock room bells went off. A man was brought in with a large portion of his brains blown out. He was slapped onto a respirator but died a few hours later. His sister and her boyfriend were brought in in the next ambulance with similar wounds. She was pronounced dead as was her boyfriend. The first patient had shot his sister and her boyfriend and then turned the gun onto himself.

In the holding area there were people on respirators. One guy was shot whilst playing dominoes at home, another was in from a terrible car crash. Few of the patients lasted more than forty-eight hours, but the respirators never had a respite. Once a patient was taken off, the plug pulled so to speak, the respirators were switched on rapidly for somebody else.

The first few weeks were interesting, I thought. I had already seen more trauma than junior doctors at home would see in a lifetime. What would the remaining weeks bring?

❖   ❖   ❖   ❖

I joined Pat the following Monday morning at seven. He wanted to put a drain or shunt from a patient's brain right down into his abdomen. This would relieve the fluid in the patient's brain which, because of scar tissue from an old bullet wound, could not drain away naturally.

We spent two-and-a-half hours putting the shunts in and I was totally flabbergasted at the amount of surgery Pat allowed me to do.

Some days later Pat showed me how to put little holes, called burr holes, in the skull bone of a patient. This was part of a craniotomy, an operation in which part of the skull is removed so that the surgeon can reach the brain underneath. I was rapidly getting used to Pat's way of teaching. He told me that the best way to learn was to watch a few operations, to assist at a few operations, then to do a few operations – under his guidance.

❖   ❖   ❖   ❖

The police were always in the accident and emergency room. They were involved in shootings and in a considerable number of cases were the victims.

Pat and myself were working on a patient one day when we noticed the sound of gunfire. Outside, the hospital grounds were crawling with 'black and whites', slang for police cars, blue lights flashing, loads of action. The gunfire was coming from the hospital roof. Two guys on the roof were shooting at anybody with a white coat. They were somewhat miffed because their mother had died in the hospital that weekend and naturally they blamed the medical staff. Luckily they did not manage to hit anybody and were coaxed down from the roof. The police could coax anything from anyone. The amount of firepower they had at their disposal, including their armoured tanks, was very persuasive.

Another afternoon I came to the door of the ER intending to do a few hours' work. The place was crawling with police, and with child-like innocence I made my way to the suture room. It was uncharacteristically empty except for one huge black man sitting on a stretcher and handcuffed to both ends. His bald head had a very nasty laceration.

Without thinking I went up to him. 'Hi,' I said. 'OK if I sew you up?'

He glanced at me quizzically and nodded.

I chatted away as I got the suture instruments ready. 'What happened to your head?'

'Pistol-whipped by the police,' he said.

I went back to work, cleaning the wound and injecting the local anaesthetic. He wanted to know where I came from as my accent was unlike anything he had ever heard before. I told him about Ireland. 'Yep, the little island near England,' and then asked him why he had been pistol-whipped.

'Blew away the family,' he said as if it was something he did every day.

I took a step backwards and looked straight into his eyes. 'Really? No kidding me?' Could I say anything else?

He told me he had 'blown away' his parents, sister and two brothers. He didn't say exactly why, but, 'They really pissed me off, Doc, you know what I mean?' He winked in a conspiratorial way.

Of course I knew, I said, it was something I came across all the time. A voice in my head screamed, Run away, run away. The man is a raving lunatic! But I stayed on and finished the job. I cut the last stitch and put the instruments down.

'All done,' I said. 'Not a bad job either.'

'Thanks, Doc, I owe you one.'

I wanted to tell him that he didn't owe me anything. Thoughts of forty years down the line came to mind, with this giant out of jail and at my door wanting to pay me back for the favour. Would I ask him to mow the lawn? Babysit the kids?

I turned to leave the room. Policemen were blocking the entrance. A sergeant came forward. 'Thanks, Doc. We thought we'd be here for hours waiting for that asshole to be sutured. Perhaps we could return the favour?'

Americans were so very friendly. First the killer and now the police wanted to do me a favour.

'Would you like to be a deputy sheriff for a day? Say next Sunday?' he asked.

I said, yes, and was told I would have to sign a disclaimer

absolving the sheriff's department of all liability in case of accident or my death. 'What are the odds?' I asked out of curiosity.

'About ten to one. Sundays are usually pretty quiet, people are sleeping off the booze and drugs from Saturday night.'

Besides my life I had nothing to lose. I accepted the invitation and looked forward to this unusual outing. As luck would have it, my bad luck of course, one of the senior staff decided to have a barbeque that Sunday and my presence was demanded. I had no choice but to get in touch with the sergeant and give my apologies. He understood my plight but, sadly, no further offers were forthcoming.

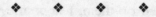

The switch from the emergency room to full-time neuro-surgical extern with Pat and Sean took about two weeks. Somebody had noticed that my general suturing and surgical technique needed a little work. I was told to report to the surgical labs. If I was unprepared for the States in general, I was completely unprepared for the surgical labs. This was where animals were operated on by medical students training to be surgeons. There were students junior to me doing dog-to-dog heart transplants. I teamed up with another student, and we went down to the dog pound and got out a huge, big, black mutt, the biggest dog there. I patted his head while the other student, who was more experienced at sneaking up on animals than I was, injected him with drugs. He went to sleep and one of the surgical technicians put a tube down his throat into his lungs, a process called intubation that keeps the patient or dog breathing.

'Now, children,' the chief surgical technician boomed. 'These there dogs need a splenectomy (removal of the spleen), a left nephrectomy (removal of the kidney), a femoral vein catherisation (sliding a tube into a vein in the leg), and a right upper lobectomy (removal of part of the lung). After that, finish him off with an intra-cardiac injection of potassium chloride.'

As I tried to remove the kidney, I nicked the aorta and the dog died in a pool of blood. We were up to our elbows in the stuff and the surgical assistant did not take kindly to our mistake. Unfortunately for the dog, it wasn't our only mistake.

I loved animals, I still do. All my life we have had cats or dogs at home, not to mention the hedgehogs, pigeons or strays that wandered into our house. I killed thirteen dogs in the two weeks I was in the States. As they were all asleep when we operated on them, I hope they did not feel any pain. I was learning all the time and in cases like this my feelings were not put on hold – they were so deeply submerged that I have never even thought about them. Killing thirteen dogs, however, is more acceptable than killing thirteen humans.

When I rejoined the neurosurgical team, Pat and Sean felt my surgical technique had improved greatly.

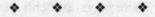

I was now assigned to the neurosurgical intensive care unit, or the NIC. The intern on neurosurgery was never around. He looked after other surgical services and had no interest in neurosurgery. While the neurosurgeons were operating there was nobody else to do the ordinary work of the unit. If I had any great difficulty there was always another doctor around. However, the NIC nurses knew more about post-op neurological cases than any junior doctor. I got on very well with them – they thought I was 'cute'! – and with their help seldom had to call any other non-neurosurgical doctors for help.

All human life and death came through the NIC doors – all those whose brains had been altered by trauma, that is. One patient named Mona got to me. She was a hooker, a junkie, one of life's losers. She had tried to take her own life but pointed the gun at the wrong part of her head. She only blew away the right frontal lobe of her brain. We operated on her, removed the bullet and brought her back to the NIC. There was no response for forty-eight hours when, suddenly, as I was holding her hand and talking to her, she squeezed my hand. I asked her to squeeze it again and she did. There were tubes everywhere, poking in and out of her but she was awake and responding. For two days we communicated by squeezing hands. She began to fight against the respirator which was a good sign.

But before we could take Mona off she got a disastrous stomach ulcer. One minute I was talking to her, the next minute blood was spewing from her mouth. We pumped her full of blood and blood expanders but she still bled. One of the general surgeons put a scope down into her stomach. There were four large ulcers. He felt that a gastrectomy (removal of her stomach) was the only answer and took her away for an emergency operation. Three hours later she was back with us. Her blood pressure started to climb and an angiogram showed that she had developed two further bleeds in her brain. That night we brought her back to the operating room, removed her right cranium and evacuated the blood that had gathered. Pat allowed me to do most of the operation.

At the end of the operation he shook his head. 'She's finished. Twenty-four hours at the most. Inform her family – if she has any.'

Mona hadn't any family. Mona had nobody. She was alone.

No visitors came to find out how she was. No flowers or get well cards. No anxious telephone calls. Mona was a nobody in the eyes of the world. I was the last person to communicate with her and when they pulled the plug the next day I was terribly upset. I was in a depression for a few days the likes of which I have never been in since. Why Mona the hooker got to me I have never figured out.

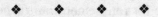

I worked very hard in neurosurgery but made time to go to other clinics of my own choice as well. My particular interest was the proctological clinic where rectal problems presented themselves. Naturally it was called the asshole clinic. My father had long ago told me if I did not stick my finger in it, I'd stick my foot in it. Off I went to the proctological clinic to do just that. The more normal rectums you examine, the more likely the chance you would find the abnormal one. But trying to convince somebody not in the procto clinic to have a rectal exam when all they have is a headache stresses the doctor/patient relationship. I examined numerous shapes, sizes and colours of bum. I felt cancers of all types, intestinal cancers, prostate cancers, haemorrhoids that were as big as grapes and anal diseases that made me wince. All in all, fantastic stuff for a medical student.

But sometimes patients made unusual requests too. One of the most unusual came when I diagnosed a large prostate gland by rectal examination on a patient who had come to have his piles attended to. The surgical resident confirmed my diagnosis. The patient stood up and asked if he could examine his own prostate gland. The resident was a little startled at the suggestion. Patients sticking their own finger up their own bum is a rarity in medicine. The resident explained that this examination was usually performed by the doctor and not by the patient. The patient responded that as it was his prostate he had every right to examine it. The resident politely told the patient what he could do with his finger and we left the cubicle.

Without blinking an eye, the patient thanked us. However, he said, he felt a second opinion was required. Whether he examined himself or not was never proved but we made sure we didn't shake his hand when he left.

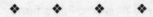

Somewhere around midway through my three months in the States I had a weekend that is etched on my mind. By now I reckoned I could help out in an emergency. I was called from the out-patients to assist at a car wreck. The victim's skull was mashed and he had a big clot pressing down on his brain. We opened him up but he died on the table. I closed the incision. Pat asked the scrub nurse to go out and tell his relatives that the patient was very badly injured but we were still operating. Ten minutes later he asked the nurse to go back to the relatives and tell them things were not looking too good. Twenty minutes later he asked the nurse to go back out again and say that nothing could be done and the surgeon would be out to tell them the worst.

'Look, John,' he said to me, 'you just can't go out and tell his closest and dearest that he's dead. You have to prepare them first. Then the surgeon goes out and informs them that he's dead.' He stood up and dropped the bombshell, 'Off you go and tell them.'

'Me? You must be joking,' I laughed in fear.

'Why not you? You're going to have to do it some day. You assisted at the operation. He was your patient, so to speak.'

'I'm a bloody medical student,' I stuttered. 'I don't tell somebody when their loved one is dead.'

'You do today,' was all he said.

My heart was thumping in my chest as I made my way to the waiting-room. I went through the doors and faced the family.

'Hello,' I said, trying to keep my voice even. I told them my name. 'I was one of the team that operated on your son. I am sorry to say that we failed to save him. I am afraid he died during the operation.' What more could I say? Here I was telling a twenty-two-year-old's family that he was dead.

I sat with them and my tears flowed with theirs. After a few minutes I stood up and shook his mother's hand. 'I am so sorry,' I whispered.

She gave me a kiss on the cheek. 'Thank you for sitting with us. Thank you for crying.'

I was devastated. I hurried out of the waiting-room and crashed into Pat. He looked at my tear-filled eyes and held me by the shoulders. 'It never gets easier, never,' he said and left me alone to regain control.

Pat was right, it never got any easier. It is the part of medicine that doctors hate most.

Night had slipped into day without us noticing it and I wanted to sleep, though I couldn't rest and my mind was buzzing. I got out of my scrub suit and went down to the ER to see what was happening. One of the shock rooms was in full use. I went in and saw an appalling injury. Gang warfare was a real problem in this city and we often saw the after effects. A young man had been shot by a rival drug gang. He had a major wound in his head and a bullet wound in his chest. The casualty doctors had opened his chest and were trying to repair the hole in his heart. There was blood everywhere. Pat came down from the operating theatre and examined the head wound. He decided that the patient was brain dead and told the other residents to stop working on his heart. I was standing right behind him and one of the residents asked me if I would like to sew up the young man's chest. His chest was open from side to side and as I put in the big sutures I could not help noticing that his heart was still beating with great force. He had exsanguinated himself (lost most of his blood), and there was nothing for the heart to pump. As I put the sutures in the heart beat slower and slower. I was putting in the last sutures when it finally shuddered and stopped.

While tidying up this patient, I heard ambulances roaring up to the hospital. There was a flurry of activity outside the other shock room and another young black male was brought in with a gunshot wound to the head. There had been a gang fight and there would be a few more ambulances. Pat was already there examining the boy who was only sixteen years old. We x-rayed him and Pat told me to prepare him for an operation to remove the bullet in his brain.

I brought the boy to the operating room with one of the ER nurses and the anaesthetist hooked him up to the necessary machines. I began to prepare his head. There was a bullet wound over the right side of his head. Brain matter was leaking out. There did not appear to be very much blood. I had covered his head with sterile drapes when Pat phoned up from the ER.

'I'll be up in a few minutes. Some more assholes have been brought in from this gang fight. Would you open his skin?'

I had done this before under supervision. I made a large incision on the right side of the boy's head, folded back the skin and put on clamps to stop the bleeding. I waited for Pat. The phone went. Over the speaker Pat asked if I had opened the skin.

'Yes.'

'OK. Can you remove the temporalis muscle and expose the skull? I'll be stuck down here for a few more minutes.'

'OK,' was all I said. I felt numb. I incised the muscle over the bullet wound using the electric cautery and exposed the skull. The wound was smaller than I had expected.

I stood back and waited. The phone went again. Pat asked what the situation was. The skull and bullet hole were exposed. Brain matter was still leaking out.

'He needs a craniectomy,' said Pat. He hesitated a few seconds. I knew what was coming. 'John, I'm in the middle of a serious problem down here. Can you nip away at the bone edge to enlarge the bullet hole for me?'

I had seen Pat 'nip' away at a few skull wounds before. I had actually 'nipped' a few myself with the surgeon beside me. I took a deep breath and asked, 'Pat, how long are you going to be?'

'Not long. Think you can do it?'

And old medical proverb says: If you can't, don't. If you can, do. I was sure I could. I had no doubt that I could remove this bullet with Pat's help.

I took a deep breath. 'Yes.'

I began to nip away at the bone and slowly enlarged the wound until I had made an area of about one square inch. Underneath lay the covering of the brain with the bullet hole right in the centre. I took a scissors and cut four straight lines through the brain coverings from the bullet hole to each side of the exposed bone. The brain lay beneath me.

'I'm not doing any more,' I said to the anaesthetist who appeared unconcerned. He gave the impression that the patient wasn't the only one inhaling the anaesthetic gases. I looked at the x-ray. The bullet was about one inch inside the brain. It seemed to be a small calibre, a Saturday Night

Special. I folded my arms and sat down on a chair.

I'm not doing any more, I thought to myself. The phone went.

'What is it like?' asked Pat.

'Not much bleeding, brain matter still leaking out, the anaesthetist says he appears stable. I'm not doing any more, Pat, I'm a bloody medical student not a neurosurgeon.'

The anaesthetist was suddenly concerned. He arched his eyebrows and peered into the wound. Then shrugging his shoulders he went back to his gases.

'I'll be up in a minute. We're nearly finished here. Listen, John, just gently remove some of the dead tissue in the hole.'

I tried to moisten my lips with my tongue. Where was my saliva? My mouth was bone dry. I stood up and asked for a forceps. I removed the pieces of dead brain that I could see. I kept on removing the tissue until I hit something hard.

Where the hell was Pat? The bullet could be resting on an artery. If I went ahead and removed it the boy could haemorrhage to death right in front of me.

Somebody was standing beside me.

'Go ahead,' said Pat softly. 'I'll look after you.'

I put the forceps into the hole and closed the points around the bullet. Sweat broke out on my forehead. Slowly I pulled the bullet out of the brain. I expected to be drenched with a torrent of blood. Nothing. I let the bullet fall into a kidney dish.

Pat looked into the hole and nodded. 'Not bad, not bad at all, Irish. Help me finish.' I assisted him in a daze.

To my delight the patient lived to fight another gun battle.

When the operation was over I was exhausted. It was now very early on Saturday morning and I went off to the rest bunks beside the OR and lay down. But my mind was racing. For the second time on that long day I could not sleep.

Exhausted as I was I could not stop thinking about what I had been allowed to do. Students were not meant to do this type of operation.

It seemed like only seconds later when an insistent ringing woke me out of a dreamless sleep.

'Hello?' I croaked into the 'phone.

'John, the place is a little nutty at the moment. Two more have come in. I need help.' It was Pat. I got up and splashed water on my face. I smelt like the bottom of a bird cage.

Down in the OR I swallowed a cup of coffee and scrubbed up. Pat was operating on a white male who had been hit on the head with a piece of wood. Unfortunately there had been a six inch nail on the end of the wood and it had gone straight into his brain. He had a skull fracture and a large inter-cerebral haematoma or clot in his brain. Pat did what was necessary, finished the operation and went into the other OR. This patient had hit his head an almighty thump on a steering wheel. When he came to us he was already paralysed on the left side with spasmodic jerking movements on his right side. He had a severe laceration in his right eye. While Pat rescrubbed I prepared the patient's head. Pat started the operation and I scrubbed up. When I got to join him I was allowed to put in the burr holes and removed the flap of bone. We eventually found the blood clot down near the base of the brain. Apparently this was a very serious problem.

'Speak to me in Irish,' Pat whispered.

'Huh?'

'Tell me some Irish sayings.'

'*Póg mo thón.*'

'What does that mean?'

'Kiss my ass.'

Pat shook with laughter. All the way through the operation I could hear Pat mumble, 'Pog muh hone, pog muh hone.'

After about an hour he stood back and scratched his back. 'OK, let's close.'

'Pog my hone, Irish,' echoed through the hospital for a few days afterwards. It must have been one of the first things our recovering patient heard when he woke up.

It was now Saturday and I had had about two hours' sleep since Friday morning. I flopped on my bed in the residency at seven o'clock that night and slept right through to the next morning – I only woke when my bladder was about to explode.

It is only *after* the rush you get with an emergency that the body – the student's or junior hospital doctor's body that is – gets exhausted. Students sometimes go for days with little or no sleep and junior hospital doctors often work up to forty-eight hours. At one operation I was watching the surgeon repair the tendons in a knife victim's wrist. I was so tired I actually fell asleep and my head fell into the wound. The surgeon was a little upset and sent me off to bed.

The doctors in the USA, especially the surgeons I met, worked *very* hard: they played hard too. Their divorce and separation rates were very high. They could not actually relax in front of the television. They had to be doing something – surgery, sports, barbeques, anything.

I was working over a hundred hours a week. I must have sutured fifteen to twenty people per day most days in my eighty-three days in the States, even when working full-time on the neurosurgical rotation. I also removed bullets, cleaned bed sores, opened abscesses and attacked anything that walked through the door. I worked so hard that I had no time to chat up any girls. Male medical students were prime targets, fair game and there were one or two attempts at relationships that never worked out, one with a nurse, the other with a beautiful black radiographer. I really hadn't the time!

❖   ❖   ❖   ❖

Still, it was not all work and no play in the States. One night Pat and I went to a party to celebrate the resignation of Richard Nixon as President of the United States.

The party was held in a teacher's house 30 miles to the north and was well on its way when we arrived. Lee, the teacher, welcomed Pat like a long-lost brother. Beer was thrust into our hands, introductions were made and we got down to the business of meeting the girls. Very soon we were extremely drunk.

I woke up in Pat's apartment the next morning. I had a terrible hangover. Pat was curled up on the floor, covered with a blanket. I was sprawled on a couch. I could see into the bedroom. The beds were untouched. Whoever had brought us home had dumped us in the sitting-room. There was a strange smell. My eyes gradually took in the state of the room. It looked as if someone had hurled a bucket of intestinal contents around. There was even some on the cactus plants. I looked at my watch. I had to clean the dial to see what time it was. Eleven o'clock on Sunday morning. I crawled over to Pat. If I looked as bad as he did we were both in serious trouble. I shook him awake and he looked at me with very suspicious eyes.

'You're a mad bastard,' he said, gagging a little.

'What did I do?' I asked innocently. My last full recollection was a tall girl telling me that she was going to the Yucatan Peninsula in Mexico the next day.

'Drunk as I was, I was not as drunk as you. On the way home in the taxi you thought we were on the wrong side of the road. You tried to get the taximan to move to the other side of the road. You were screaming that the driver was trying to kill us. I had to restrain you from leaping over the seat. You can imagine how pleased the driver was especially when I asked him to help carry you into the apartment.' He appeared to hesitate.

'And?' I prompted.

'You puked up all over his shoes.' I nodded in understanding and pointed to some little pools of dry material.

'... the plants, the floor, the couch, me. Luckily the cat was out.'

'All mine?' I asked.

'Well, not exactly. That on the floor near the stairs is mine.'

So I wasn't totally to blame. I crawled back to the couch indifferent now to the mess. I slept for another few hours. When I woke up Pat was making a bacon sandwich. The smell hit my stomach like an invading army. This time I made it to the toilet.

❖   ❖   ❖   ❖

My last week in early September was a blur of activity, but one marathon operation stands out. I called over to the ER one afternoon and was told that Pat was in the OR doing a laminectomy, that is removing the backbone, on a young man. Expecting the junior resident to be there I went to have a look. Medical students at home had little opportunity to see this type of operation which exposed the actual spinal cord. I poked my head around the door.

Pat caught sight of me. 'Wash your hands, John.' And that was that.

The operation was on a twenty-three-year-old who had been complaining of progressive upper extremity weakness for about six months. We removed the backbone from the skull to the middle of his back. There was a large evil-looking cancer in his spinal cord. Huge veins were draining the cancer and it was inoperable. One of the senior staff neurosurgeons was called in and did a bit of poking around. He left after about fifteen minutes. Pat took a tiny piece of the tumour away for pathological examination. It confirmed the cancer. We finished the operation nine hours after starting. Surgically, nothing could be done for the poor guy. Pat reckoned he had about six months before the tumour caught up with him.

❖　　　❖　　　❖　　　❖

Before I left the States, Pat gave a small party in his apartment. Small, but very rowdy. Feeling a little low, I said my goodbyes to my new friends.

I arrived home in Dublin. I had never worked with the famous cardiac surgeon. But it didn't matter. I wanted to be a neurosurgeon. I had done more than I had ever dreamt possible for a medical student. I had taken a bite of the surgical big apple which was wonderful. I had got my hands bloody, I had delved into the innards of the human brain, and to top it off, the chairman of the neurosurgical department had offered me a place in neurosurgical training when my studies in Ireland were finished. All heady stuff! Two years later I was in the Massachusett's General Hospital in Boston on neurosurgical extern rotation. But more of that later.

Chapter 4

Third Med

*R*eal medicine at long last! As Third Med students, we were assigned to hospital rotations which meant spending some weeks with various specialties and watching the senior hospital doctors and consultants deal with the problems they were the experts in solving. Along with this were lectures in Microbiology, Pathology, Pharmacology, Social and Preventative Medicine and Forensic Medicine. I had learned how the body worked, now I had to learn what happened when something went wrong. Beating diseases was as yet something in the future.

Pathology was one of the more important subjects. The lectures were by and large very interesting. They were generally in the early afternoons and if anybody had had a liquid lunch they could be found at the back of the auditorium snoring contently. One of the lecturers like to spice up his slides of diseased organs with slides of his family holidays. Without warning, a slide of his happy family in some exotic location would appear just after a picture of a stomach tumour or such like. We got to know his family quite well. These diversions endeared this teacher to the class. He unfortunately had the less liked habit of giving out wrong tips for exams. We learned from more senior classes that whatever tips he gave out were sure *not* to be on the paper. He actually became a patient of mine some years later.

One of the lecturers in Microbiology was an old friend of my father's. His lectures were always fun. He had a biting wit that helped us to get through the lectures on Staphylococcus, Neisseria, Streptococcus, Ecoli and many more bugs that we would come to know and love. One or two of my classmates would even get acquainted with Neisseria gonococci – a form of VD on a more personal level.

However, it was a more senior member in one of the disciplines in medicine who was infamous. He was, to be nice about it, eccentric. He invented an apparatus to test the balancing mechanism in the inner ear. This apparatus was no more than a swing that could do a complete 360% circle. He would ask for volunteers to test it and, thinking that by volunteering their chances in the examinations would be enhanced, somebody would always volunteer. The unfortunate student would sit on the swing and the lecturer would push him or her until the swing was doing the 360% circle. Quite a few got sick. Watching one of your colleagues hurtling around on the contraption, spewing out his lunch was, of course, a source of endless amusement to the rest of us. Our lecturer also liked to sit students in a chair that turned a full circle. This also had a tendency to upset the balancing mechanisms in the ear with the similar result that the stomach's contents were violently voided. He also arranged the oral examinations so that many students would be examined at night. He would inform many students in front of the class that their papers were 'rubbish' or 'crap'. But he was fair in exams and that was important to us.

Pharmacology was about drugs and their effects on living tissue. We had animals to take the brunt of the tests as none of us volunteered to sample the choice of chemicals. Rabbits were the most popular choice, followed by cats and dogs. A few students freed some of the rabbits and the police were called. They were somewhat bewildered to be called by the School of Pharmacology and refused to go chasing the rabbits all over the fields.

We tested dogs with morphine and watched as the morphine took effect. The dogs puked all over the place. Not so the cats. It was fascinating to watch as after a shot of morphine a docile cat turned into a mad moggy – spitting, hissing and charging around the classroom. However instructive this was, giving morphine to animals is not something I have come across in general practice very often.

Forensic Medicine dealt with the legal side of medicine, especially accidental death, murder and suicide. These lectures were usually attended by students from other faculties who had heard about the grisly pictures and slides that were shown. Lectures in Pathology had prepared us medical students somewhat for these picture shows, but not so the engineering students who would come up from the faculty in Merrion Row or the architects who inhabitated the same part of the university as we did. As slides of bodies and what had happened to them were projected on screen, groans followed by thumps could be heard from the non-medics in the lecture theatre. To this day I believe that the professors knew when the non-medics were in the class and showed the most sickening pictures on purpose.

One of the more bizarre stories we heard was of a forensic pathologist called down to the country some years ago where a mummified body had been dug up in a bog. The doctor hadn't brought the necessary instruments with him so he had to drive back to Dublin for them. When he returned, the body was gone. The locals had descended en masse during the night and had cut up the body for holy relics. They thought that, because there was a monastery near by, the preserved body was that of a saint.

We were also taught that suicide did not always work. The lecturer in Forensics told us of a famous case of a depressed person who knew exactly what he wanted to do. He lived near a cliff and so built a gallows out over the raging surf. He put his neck in the noose, swallowed a lot of pills, and shot himself in the head while he was hanging himself. The bullet bounced off his temple, cut through the rope and he fell into the sea. He swallowed a bucketful of salt water which made him vomit up all the pills he had taken. He swam ashore with only a small graze on his head, admitted himself to the local hospital and lived a full and happy life.

As the year progressed we spent more and more time in hospital. Half the class went to the Mater and half went to St Vincent's Hospital. I was a resident student in St Vincent's and actually lived in the hospital residence. A salary was way in the future but, as consolation, we could see the nurses' home on the other side of the hospital. And though we could not get through the security at the front door of the nurses' home, let alone into the rooms, they could get into the residency. Impromptu parties were arranged on many nights across in the Merrion Inn, our local watering hole, and cause of many a sore head – the place was fondly known as MI: myocardial infarction, or heart attack. This was a useful codeword which could be used when a thirst descended in the middle of a ward round.

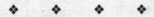

We had to take hospital rounds with an air of professionalism at this stage. As resident students we were supposed to know most of the patients.We were allowed to listen to hearts, percuss chests, feel abdomens and generally prod and poke the patients for as long as they could stand it. The interns, the lowest possible grade of doctor, were usually too busy to teach us. We were stuck with senior house officers (SHOs) and the doctors who actually ran a department, the registrars. Above the registrars were the senior registrars, doctors who were waiting for a consultant's post. Finally, at the top of the pile came the consultant, the main man, El Supremo, the rich one. All, of course, were subservient to the ward sister. Mixed with this imposing bunch of medical knowledge were research registrars, special lecturers and tutors. On rounds, when we went from bed to bed examining patients – there could be up to ten white-coated individuals, as well as the ward sisters, ward staff nurses and the student nurses.

On one of our first rounds we came to a mildly confused woman who had projectile vomiting, a sign that all was not well with her intestines. A surgical registrar was trying to ask her to describe the problem. She was having a little bit of difficulty understanding the question and was somewhat nervous of the ten white-coated doctors around her bed. She hummed and hawed.

One of the students could take it no longer. He stepped forward, and in a broad country accent, asked: 'Tell me, Missus, does your puke hit the wall when you vomit?'

We expected her to be shocked. She nodded her head vigorously.

'Why yes,' she beamed. 'It actually frightened the dog once.'

The registrar sniffed, coughed, said thank you and we carried on to the next bed.

In another ward there was a female patient of about eighteen years of age who had a fractured leg. She was very popular with the interns as she insisted on injections in her buttocks. One of the other students and I were at the end of the bed with our hands resting on the bed itself. The orthopaedic registrar proceeded to tell us how the accident happened. He put the plate into her broken leg and asked her to lift her leg to show how mobile it now was. A demonstration like this may sometimes be a little tedious. Not this time. The young beauty had no pants on under the short nightie! I stood bolt upright and whimpered. The other student was transfixed. As yet we had not developed a mature outlook on girls, especially those without pants. We were the only two to see what was going on while she was flinging her leg around in wild abandon, the only students who were sweating, with stupid grins on their faces. Maybe she didn't realise she had no knickers on. After the story got around, she was besieged by male students wanting to examine her leg from the end of the bed instead of from the side.

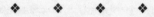

Our time in residency in St Vincent's coincided with our finding the 'reading room'. This room became a safe haven for a group of about thirteen of us. We used to study there until we did our final examinations. The thirteen of us also tended to hang around together all through Med School. I suppose, with the wonder of hindsight, I could say we were the rowdies of the hospital. Anybody who smoked, drank and chased the opposite sex was welcome at the reading room. And it was there that I came to know my future medical partner, Paddy Duggan, warts and all. The reading room was where we could sleep off a hangover rather than actually study, an occupation which to the reading room student was particularly rare. Those who really wanted to study did so in the hospital library.

Each university year lasted about forty weeks of which the

last six weeks of the year before exams were days of intensive study often lasting up to eighteen hours. These brain-busting episodes got us all through the exams with the occasional hiccup. It was ironic that whilst only one of the reading room students failed the final exam, two of the library students went down.

It was in the reading room that we were observed examining one of our colleague's testicles. As preparation for the exams, we would study each other's medical problems. I had a funny noise in my chest that was examined by the others. Another student was a sportsman with early arthritis in his left hip. This was examined as well. When one of the others explained that he had a little collection of blood vessels on his testicle called a varicocele, we just had to have a look, girls and all.

The large windows of the reading room looked out onto one of the walks where the hospital nuns used to say their prayers. We moved some coat rails around so the student with the odd ball would be hidden from prying eyes. We gathered around him with great expectation. He dropped his trousers and underpants dutifully and we bent down to inspect the offending testicle. Somebody stumbled and the coat rail was pushed over. At that moment one of the hospital nuns was showing three visiting nuns the walks outside the reading room. They were also given a very clear view of a crowd of students watching, and some actually examining, the testicle of another student. All he said was, 'Uh oh!'

We spun around to see four pale faces outside the window. The nuns' eyes were out on stalks. They appeared to be shrieking – the glass was double-glazed so thankfully we could not hear the noise. They ran towards the convent, glancing behind them as if the student with the exposed gonads was chasing them.

We went back to our studies. Suddenly the reading room door was flung open and a senior nun burst in like a witch. She had never had a testicle examined in her reading room before!

'You crowd of filth!' she thundered. 'How dare you expose the nuns to such scenes. You must be the rowdiest, the worst mannered, the dirtiest band of . . . '

The door had been caught in the breeze and banged shut. She couldn't continue. She was struck speechless by what she saw next. 'Miss December' was plastered on the back of the door!

'I think she's going to have a heart attack,' said one of the girls. 'Who's going to do the mouth to mouth?'

With a theatrical 'Humph!' the nun whipped open the door and left us a little shocked. One of the girls said, 'We'll either be sent to nursing school or booted out. Or she may be too embarrassed to say a word. Let's go to the happy hour.'

Our 'happy hour' was from five to seven in a hotel close to the hospital. The cheapest drink was an Irish coffee made from what we reckoned was Nigerian whiskey. At one of these sessions, ten of us managed to consume a hundred-and-thirty-one Irish coffees. That same night one of the participants tried to drive his car through casualty. The porter lost control of his bladder when he saw the Morris Minor hurtling through the doors. But he sprang into action. He was only a tiny little man but he stood in front of the car.

'Get that thing out of here, you little gobshite!' he shouted over the roar of the engine as he tried to push the car out. He got the two fingers from the student.

'Right! That's it. You're on report to the night matron.' Being on report to the night matron, the hospital boss, was on the same level as a rectal exam – unpleasant.

Before the student had any chance of gasing anybody with

the exhaust, the car shot backwards out of the casualty to hide behind the hospital.

This Morris Minor was famous in its own right. The student who owned it tended to lose his money in poker so could not afford a flat. He lived in his car. Every morning his consultant surgeon would knock on the car roof and wake him up. A groggy-eyed, unwashed head would poke out of the window, mumble and disappear into the car again. A few hours later the car would be aired when the student finally crawled out and joined his team.

Chapter 5

Fourth Med

There was no long summer break between Third and Fourth Med. They melted into each other with only the exams to divide them.

We were now allowed to examine and interview patients and we presented the patient to the consultant and the rest of the team on ward rounds. However well prepared we were for the illness, we could not be prepared for what the patient said.

Perhaps it was my father who prepared me for some of my more unusual meetings with patients in my early career. He told me that when he was a casualty officer many years ago, a woman had brought her child into the casualty with a sore penis. The child was very frightened and refused to budge. My father showed remarkable calmness when the women said in a warm Dublin accent, 'Show the doctor your willy and he'll kiss it better.'

Genitalia featured much in misunderstandings. During my Paediatric rotation I was in casualty when a worried mother brought her seven-year-old son in. The casualty officer asked me to examine the child.

'He's got a lump on his mickey,' his mother said, gazing down on her nearest and dearest.

'His penis,' I said with great authority. 'He has a lump on his penis.'

'Never mind that lump, have a look at this mickey.'

As gently as I could I removed the boy's trousers and inspected the little member. There was something odd about the lump under his foreskin. It appeared to be quite sticky. I removed it very easy between my index finger and my thumb.

'What's that?' his mother enquired.

'Chewing gum,' I replied. Little boys are very curious. Why not shove a piece of chewing gum into your willy? So are men. As a casualty officer in a northside hospital, I once had to remove a toothpaste tube from an adult patient's rectum.

On my gynaecology rotation I was totally confused when a sweet young thing told me that she had a problem with wind.

'Perhaps you need to see a stomach specialist,' I said.

'But I'm farting through my fanny. What good is a belly man?'

What good indeed? I thought. On examination by the consultant, he found she had a problem between her rectum and vagina and needed an operation to repair it.

❖   ❖   ❖   ❖

Between November and January my fellow students and I attended twenty-two parties, mostly given by friends. Some we gate-crashed.

We heard that there was to be a fancy dress party in one of the other hospitals. I borrowed one of my mother's old white bathing suits, made a pair of wings and halo out of cardboard and silver foil and topped off the costume with a very flimsy nightgown. I couldn't find a pair of shoes in my size to complement the outfit and so wore a pair of army boots instead. I arrived at the hospital and burst in through the door into the party.

There is a significant difference between 'dress party' and a 'fancy dress party' I discovered. Everybody else was in dress suits and very expensive gowns. I was dressed as a fairy godmother in army boots. It was a party for the senior hospital staff, all of whom were looking at me.

One of the consultants came over. 'Perhaps you're at the wrong party, young lady – or whatever you are.'

'I'm a fairy godmother,' I whispered.

'And very fetching you are.' He turned to the other people in the room. 'Friends and colleagues, our fairy godmother has arrived.'

There were cheers and applause and I was invited to stay for a drink.

A few weeks later I won a prize at a real fancy dress party wearing the same outfit. The prize was a cosmetics set for the best-dressed woman.

❖   ❖   ❖   ❖

In January I decided to leave home. Residency was over for the moment and I would have to move back to my parent's house. However, some of my friends had moved into a house near the hospital and I felt a need to join them. When I left home my parents told their friends that I had run away.

The other students in the house were two friends from the reading room and an accountancy student. For all my messing about I was very regimented when it came to getting up in the morning. No matter how blitzed I had been the night before I would force myself out of bed. The other three had a mental block about the mornings. I would get up at eight and call them. After breakfast I would call them again. If I got back to the house at lunchtime I would call them again. It was usually about three o'clock before they finally arose.

Luckily we were attending a hospital dealing with psychiatric patients and the staff were never sure how many students were supposed to attend, let alone their names. In the eight weeks I spent in the house we had only one party and I lost about a stone in weight, eating whatever was left by the mice. Bowing to the inevitable – and the hunger pains – I went back to my folks. They could have been happier.

The class was beginning to settle down to study as the finals were only one summer away. Parties were now seriously interrupted by lectures, clinics and tutorials. We were beginning to get the feel of looking after patients and to watch with interest their day-to-day care.

Casualty was one of the places where we could practise our new-found techniques, especially on the drunks who were anaesthetised anyway. My few months in the USA were invaluable to me here. I could take blood, set up IVs, suture patients, help at cardiac arrests and generally make myself useful. My skills in the neurosurgical field were not required, much to my disquiet. It was also a disappointment to find that the trauma in casualty was not as varied as that in America.

I was the casualty student on call one Saturday when a sailor walked in with what appeared to be rectal bleeding. He was put on a stretcher and asked to drop his trousers. He lay on his stomach and from what he told me it sounded like he had a case of haemorrhoids. He was big, smelly and unwashed – I thought it prudent to let the doctor examine him. The casualty officer that night was a rather solemn, tall, muscle-bound rugby player who appeared to me to take life far too seriously. He strolled into the cubicle and asked what the problem was.

'I think he has haemorrhoids,' I said.

'Did you examine him?' he asked.

I smiled and mouthed, 'You must be joking.'

The doctor put on a stalk (a plastic sheath that pulls over the doctor's finger), smeared it with KY jelly and asked the sailor to spread his legs a little so he could examine his bum. Patients' rectums are normally examined when they are lying on their left side, but the casualty officer's method was a little different.

This I had to see. Large unwashed buttocks were pulled apart and the injured part was examined. The doctor now had his left arm resting on the patient's left shoulder and his right index finger halfway up his rectum. Another student came in and in a friendly manner put his right hand on the patient's right shoulder. The patient had been very quiet up until this moment. His head came up like lightning from the pillows. As far as he was concerned he was being buggered by the doctor. He let out a strangled roar and leapt off the stretcher. This sudden contraction of his buttocks created a sucking effect on the finger-stalk and pulled it off the doctor's finger. The patient stood wide-eyed in the main casualty area, a little out of place with no trousers on and a long plastic finger-stalk hanging out of his bum like a cow's udder. He pointed an accusing finger at the doctor.

'He tried to bugger me,' he screamed at the staff nurse.

The doctor was a little confused. He held his finger in the air looking around for the little finger stalk.

'If you just calm down, sir, I am sure we can work this out,' the staff nurse said in a calm friendly voice.

One of the student nurses came around the corridor, saw the patient and pointed at the finger-stalk dangling from his anus. The patient opened his legs and bent down to have a look. He looked through his legs, past the dangling finger-stalk and into the full waiting-room, usually full of bedlam and noise. Not now. Everybody had suspended whatever he or she was doing and was transfixed by the sight.

Full marks must be given to the patient at this point. Not only did he think that he had met a gay doctor but now he had exposed his anus to total strangers.

He stood up calmly and without hesitation slowly extracted the finger-stalk. He walked over to the doctor and slapped it into his hand, closing the doctor's fingers over the stalk so that it made a squelching noise.

'Oh yuck!' said the student nurse.

❖ ❖ ❖ ❖

While on the casualty rotation, I found that patients would confide in you if they thought you were a doctor. The white coat was a signal to unburden their problems and not just medical problems.

When asked his occupation one patient said: 'I'm a burglar.'

'You're a what?' I asked incredulously.

'I'm a burglar. I rob houses. That's how I make my living.'

He seemed such a nice man, I thought, and noted his address just to make sure he was not living too close to home.

Another time I was just going off-duty when I caught sight of a long graceful leg dangling over the side of a stretcher in a cubicle. I like to think it was professional curiosity that led me to the cubicle. My heart told me I had to find out where that long slender leg ended and who owned it. A heavily made-up 'lady of the night' was lying on the stretcher. She was a little drunk. I was about to leave when she caught my coat.

'Hello, big boy,' she whispered in a poor imitation of a French accent. She sounded as if she came from Cork and had had her throat cut. I backed off a little.

'Fancy a little freebee, maybe?' She giggled to herself.

Perhaps some of my colleagues who would have taken up the offer, flung her to the floor, drunk or not, and would have made enough noise to alert the police. But I shook my head and thanked her for the kind offer. It was against hospital rules for the student staff to bonk the patients. I believe it still is.

❖   ❖   ❖   ❖

It was now late spring and we were studying for our finals in the minor subjects, Eyes, Ear, Nose and Throat Surgery and Psychiatry. I *had* to pass the exams as I had already booked a flight to spend the summer in Boston, doing *what* I had yet to decide.

All too soon the exams were on us. The ENT (Ear, Nose and Throat) exam was composed of a clinical exam and an oral exam. The child I had to examine had a simple chronic ear complaint that should have presented me with no problem. He was about nine years old and would not let me near him. I tried to bribe him with a bag of sweets. Finally I whispered that I would wring his bloody neck if he did not let me examine him. He appeared to get the message.

The oral was next. I came into the room where the two examiners sat behind a desk. They motioned me to sit down.

'You did very well in the clinical examination,' the senior consultant said.

'Thank you, sir,' I replied.

'A difficult little lad, that one. He was very restless with some of the other students.'

'I have a way with children, sir.'

'Good, good. Now tell me what you know about recurrent laryngeal palsy in children.'

'I beg your pardon?' I thought he had cursed at me.

'Yes, vocal chord paralysis in children, due to a dysfunction in the recurrent laryngeal nerve.'

How could he keep a straight face, I wondered, asking a student a question like that? I had never heard of this problem in children. I had never even read about it in the books.

'Well,' I stammered. 'Paralysis of the vocal chords in children is not very common. I would expect that they would present with persistent hoarseness.'

There was a knock on the door and another examiner came into the room. They discussed another case for a few moments and then turned back to me.

'Sorry about the interruption. Now where were we?'

'You were asking me about hoarseness in children,' I blurted out.

'Oh really? Tell me about the common causes of hoarseness then.'

Off I went. I did very well in the ENT exam.

A few days later we had our Psychiatry exam in St Brendan's Hospital, the main mental hospital in Dublin. First we watched two video-taped interviews with patients. The first video was about a paranoid schizophrenic, the second video was about a patient with a peculiar personality disorder. The students from our reading room felt a great sympathy with this one.

When the show was over we bombarded the brighter students about what we had seen. I put down as much information as I could on a sheet of paper and tried to memorise it before I was interrogated by the examiners. When I was called into the examiners to answer questions on the tapes, I stuck the paper into my jacket pocket. I knocked on the door.

'Come in. Sit down. Relax,' said one of the examiners. I

think he thought I was a patient.

'Now, using whatever information you have, tell me about the second case you watched on the video.'

It was make or break time I thought. The phrase 'using whatever information you have' was like a light at the end of a very dark tunnel. I swallowed hard and took out the sheet of paper that I had stuck into my pocket.

'I wrote down some information during the film,' I said. 'Could I refer to it while answering your questions?'

'Why not,' said the psychiatrist.

I quoted verbatim what I had written down about the patient with the personality disorder. I was not at all surprised that I gathered a second class honour. Actually most students that day got a second class honour.

I had passed my minor finals. Celebrations were called for and myself and my reading room pals duly took over the Ballsbridge Inn – or the BBI as it was fondly known. The rest of the night is a happy, foggy memory.

❖   ❖   ❖   ❖

America – The Second Trip

My friends from the reading room went to Boston a week before I did to fix up an apartment. They knew the lie of the land as they had been there on previous summers. A very good friend of mine was a pilot and he arranged it so that I could fly to Boston via New York with the crew – the fulfilment of a long-held ambition!

My friend pre-boarded me on to the Boeing 707 and sat me in the navigator's seat in the cockpit behind him. As I was an honorary member of the flight crew I had to make sure that the oxygen mask assigned to me was working. I put it on and flicked down the check switches to test the oxygen was coming through. At that precise moment a medical student from the year below me came into the cockpit to have a look. He looked at me in astonishment – a medical student apparently working with the crew.

He could not contain himself. 'Hey!' he blurted out. 'You're not a pilot.'

'Day job,' I boasted.

He backed away, terror in his face. A medical student was up in the cockpit helping to fly the plane!

When we arrived in New York a few hours later, I learnt that Boston was fogbound. I met up with four other people trying to get to Boston. We decided to rent a car and split the bill. I was dropped at a hotel in Boston as I had no idea where my apartment was. I went in and booked a room for the night for twelve dollars.

'Anything else needed?' asked the male receptionist.

'No thanks,' I said. 'Why?'

He looked around and raised his eyebrows. I looked

around as well. There were a few ladies sitting around the place.

'Things are quiet. Thirty dollars a night. Twenty dollars if you go with one of the older ones,' he said with a leer.

I declined for two reasons: I was knackered and I had only ten dollars on me.

I phoned my friends the next morning. When they came to collect me one of them expressed a desire to stay at the hotel. We set off back to our apartment and my friends filled me in on things. The apartment was situated on the wrong end of Commonwealth Avenue, and the job situation did not appear to be good. We told Immigration that we were on a three-month holiday and produced letters to show that we could support ourselves for that length of time. We actually had enough money for about ten days. We were over on holiday visas and were breaking the law by working.

Our first week was spent in Cape Cod celebrating the bicentenary of American Independence. We invaded a local pub with our new girlfriends and entertained the locals with an on-stage performance. One of the girls, a very strange nurse from Massachusett's General Hospital, brought the house down with what she called the Epileptic Shuffle. She would collapse on the stage and twitch around, ending with a very acceptable imitation of frothing at the mouth. She was asked back the following night but, unfortunately, we had to look for work. We had heard that one of the numerous security firms springing up in Boston around that time was looking for Irish students. The Irish had a reputation for honesty and hard work. In other words we could be trusted.

Another student and I walked for miles before we finally found the security firm. The interview was quick and to the point.

'You Irish students?' asked the manager. He glared at our

passports. 'Ever own a gun? Ever in jail? Ever use dope? You're hired.'

We were given uniforms and told to report for duty the following Monday. In fact, we were nothing more than porters, without the tips. People signed in and people signed out. The building housed various offices: a bar school, psychologists, tax experts, a sexologist and a fashion model agency. Some of the girls who walked past my desk were straight from the pages of a fashion magazine. They didn't even glance at me until I decided to bring in some of my medical books to pass the time.

One of the girls asked me for change for the public telephone. She noticed my text books.

'You a Pre-Med student?'

'I finish Medical School next year,' I said matter-of-factly.

Her eyes lit up. For obvious reasons medical students were looked upon as treasure chests and were hunted down without mercy. I could almost see the dollar signs over my head. All she said was, 'Really?' and my life changed dramatically.

One of my security duties was to check out a very fashionable ladies' club. I would arrived at about eight o'clock and walk through the whole building. The telephonist's board was not to be used, but as I had worked as a telephonist in a medical deputising service some years before, I figured out the contraption on my second night. I could now phone whoever I wanted. This, along with the ladies from the modelling school, made my stay in Boston more bearable.

One weekend I happened to pass the Massachusett's General Hospital which is famous for its high medical standards. It was and is a famous teaching hospital and research institution. It was there that the first successful public demonstration of surgical anaesthesia was performed in 1846. The theatre where this was carried out is preserved as a historical site. My father had written *The History of Medicine in Ireland*, and I looked forward to telling him I had seen it. It would be a real feather in my cap to get a job there. How this came about was unusual to say the least.

❖   ❖   ❖   ❖

An Irish consultant held a party one night. His brother was in our mob and so we were all invited. Six of us arrived at the consultant's home and were immediately surrounded by the Secret Service. We knew they were Secret Service because they were talking into their buttonholes and sported large revolvers in their armpits. We were not to know that an Irish politician was at the party. It was the mid-seventies and the Secret Service was worried about the IRA. They must have shit daisies rectally when we arrived on the scene.

'Stay-in-the-car. Do-not-move. Stay-in-the-car,' a staccato voice ordered. One of the men came over cautiously to the car.

'Is one of you Donal, the brother of Patrick?'

Donal nodded. The light was shone into our faces. Unblinking eyes scanned us slowly and finally we were allowed in. The Irish politician was drunk. He had already vomited and had become something of an embarrassment. Maybe we were getting old but we thought that as a representative of our country he was a very poor choice.

Someone introduced me to an Irish ENT surgeon who was a senior resident in Massachusett's General Hospital. By the end of the evening I had myself a job in neurosurgery. On a Saturday morning at seven o'clock the phone rang and I was told to present myself for an interview in an hour's time in the Professor of Neurosurgery's office. We had gone to bed at five o'clock with a load of cold beer on board, but I wanted the name of Massachusett's General Hospital on my CV.

The professor asked me where I had worked before. I told him about my previous work in the States and I told him about Pat. There and then he picked up the phone and phoned him. The professor asked if he remembered an Irish medical student named John from two years before.

'Sure, I remember John,' I could hear Pat say. That was it. I was in. All I had to do was to enrol in the Harvard Medical School and become a neurosurgical extern.

I did my neurosurgical rotation from eight in the morning to four in the afternoon. But to be blunt, it was not the same game as before. There were no gunshot wounds, no decapitations, no brains all over the accident and emergency room. All the surgery was cold – not an emergency – and was pre-arranged by the consultant who had diagnosed the problem. It was not until a few weeks later that I found out I should have gone to one of the trauma hospitals.

I was introduced to the Cuban resident named Raoul and his junior resident, Tom. Neither appeared enthusiastic at the prospect of having a foreign student on their team. Naturally I cultivated outside interests to keep my mind off the job.

After my day in neurosurgery was over, I would turn up for my security job. This was a doddle until the afternoon one of the apartment residents came into the foyer.

'Hey you!' he pointed at me. 'You're the security guard?'

I nodded.

'There are some guys in the office block next door. You better throw them out.'

I looked over my shoulder to make sure that there wasn't a big, burly, gun-toting security guard standing behind me.

'Me?' I asked.

He nodded.

'Bugger off and call the police.'

'You're the security guard. Put them out,' he insisted.

In my mind's eye I saw myself sailing out through a window about ten storeys up.

'If you think I'm going to put my ass in a sling for you, you must be out of your mind,' I replied.

He literally dragged me to the elevator and pushed me in. 'Now, run them out of this building.'

I started to laugh. 'And what would I use?' I was getting a little excitable.

'What about your gun?' The light was dawning on him slowly.

'I don't have a gun. I don't have a knife, a night stick. I have nothing. Shall I tie them up with my shoelaces?' I don't normally use bad language. I did then. I think I made him more scared of me than he was of the intruders. At one point I was actually spitting at him.

When I finally found the nerve to go next door the building was empty.

❖   ❖   ❖   ❖

One of my roommates had a job in a bar. Naturally we invited ourselves for a few free beers more than once. On one occasion our roommate was pulling pints with an uncharacteristically wild look in his eyes. At the back of the bar a hooker was leaning against an old jukebox, winking at him. Usually the bar closed at around two in the morning. Not tonight.

'Right! All out, the bar is closed,' he said, his agitation obvious.

Luckily there was only a dozen or so of us in the bar that night. We poured out of the pub. One of the female guests was missing. From inside the bar there was a noise like two express trains meeting. The building seemed to shake. The shouts and screams emanating from inside were unlike anything I had ever heard before or since. I thought somebody was bound to call the police. Ten minutes later the doors were opened by a much calmer roommate and we were allowed back in. Drinks were on the house. On one of the seats lay someone who looked like she had been run over by an elephant!

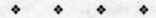

My surgical rotation in Massachusett's General was turning out to be a little disappointing. I watched numerous procedures but 'hands on' time was very limited. The only enjoyable surgical moments were with a famous neurosurgeon named Dr John Ballintine. He had written text books on the subject and was recognised as one of the world's best neurosurgeons. I met him by accident when I wandered into the operating room.

'Would you like to scrub with me, young man?' he asked gently.

I liked him immediately. I scrubbed up and joined him at the operating table. He was about to take a piece of bone from a patient's hip and put it into the patient's spine, an operation called a spinal fusion. He took the bone out and dropped it into some salt solution in a kidney dish. He began to open the back. He turned and looked at me.

'Would you mind suturing the hip, please?' he asked.

I was a bit taken aback. I could crack a skull open, but a hip? He thought I was a resident in surgery.

'I'm a student, Dr Ballintine,' I said. 'My knowledge of surgery is somewhat limited.'

He nodded and enquired how much experience I had had. I told him briefly about my time in the States.

'I'll show you what to do then you can carry on, OK?'

I assisted him on several occasions after that. Dr Ballintine was one of life's gentlemen and it was an honour to have known him.

❖　　❖　　❖　　❖

In the mid-seventies, CAT scanners, a special form of x-ray imaging, were very much a rarity. Ireland had none, but everyone was talking about them. I got to see one of the first in the x-ray department in Mass General. The radiologists went to great lengths to show me amazing photographs of the brain. I decided to spend a few days there watching this new technique and met another well-known neurosurgeon who invited me to assist him. His forte was the very painful condition known as trigeminal neuralgia in which a cranial nerve from the brain causes excruciating pain in the face. The cause is unknown but this surgeon had developed a technique that destroyed the nerve as it left the skull. Apart from Dr Ballintine, he was the only surgeon who allowed me to do some of the operations.

My earlier experience in the States perhaps made me big-headed but I was not content just to stand and do nothing at an operation. I began to change my mind about a career in neurosurgery. I had great fun as a security guard with the fashion models, I had seen the sights of Boston and assisted famous surgeons, but I felt unhappy. I felt I had arrived at a significant juncture in my medical life. It was make-my-mind-up-time career-wise and neurosurgery was not as appealing as I had once thought. I decided to cut short my stay in Boston.

One of my sisters, Caroline, married a GP in London, Ontario. During my first few weeks in Boston it was Tony, my sister's husband, who sent down the occasional few bucks just to keep myself and my friends from starving. My parents were visiting my sister and I decided to join them. I took a Trailways bus to London – an eighteen-hour journey but cheap, and arrived in the middle of the night. I was totally knackered. My bawdy days were apparently catching up on me.

A few days later my family and I were invited to a party given by a radiologist who lived nearby. I had far too much to drink and my father decided to walk me home. Some things stick in your mind no matter how inebriated you are. I stumbled on the footpath, and my father steadied me by putting his arm around my shoulders.

In that split second I had made up my mind to forget neurosurgery.

'Dad, I want to be a GP,' I said.

He nodded with the greatest of understanding and said, 'We'll talk about it in the morning.'

The rest of my holidays was spent relaxing and sunbathing. In my subconscious I was getting ready for the finals. I had got this far, nothing was going to stop me from becoming a doctor. I even looked forward to restarting my studies – a very unusual frame of mind for me.

Chapter 6
Final Med

Final Med consisted of Surgery, Medicine, Obstetrics, Gynaecology and Paediatrics. One of my stints in Ob/Gyn, as we called Obstetrics and Gynaecology, started at the time of the party season. One or other had to suffer. The parties were especially good that year but the Ob/Gyn rotation interfered in a big way and I had to study. I had to get down to it. Ob/Gyn clinics, where we learned how to do gynaecological examinations, were held nearly every day. If I attended even two out of three clinics I would learn all I needed to pass the exam.

We medical students initially felt awkward when it came to female examinations. I personally felt more embarrassment for the patient than myself, for, no matter how you handled the procedure, she had to allow you to carry out an examination that was a little unpleasant.

My rotation in the delivery room brought me face to face with new babies. I watched a few being born before I was assigned my own patient who was on her tenth delivery. She was a tough, rough woman who fired out babies like bullets. During her labour the midwife left for a few seconds.

'It's coming! It's coming! The baby is on the way!' the woman shouted.

'Come on, you,' she pointed at me. 'Deliver the little bastard!'

With the knowledge I had gathered from watching other births I began to assist the birth.

The patient lifted her head up and squinted at me. 'You're new at this, aren't you?'

I nodded. 'Relatively.'

She actually sat up and peered down between her legs. 'Here, this is how it's done.' She got hold of my hands and put them on the baby's head which had now appeared. 'You pull, while I push.'

What could I say? It was her tenth baby, she knew more about it than I did. The baby exploded out of her like a wet rugby ball.

New babies are very slippery and ugly. This one looked like a troll. I fumbled with this human rugby ball and held him upside down to drain the mucus from his mouth.

'Nurse, Nurse!' the patient shouted. 'He's going to drop it!'

The baby took a deep breath and let out a roar.

Bloody hell, I thought, I've delivered a baby. I looked down at the human troll and saw that his blue skin was turning a healthy pink. Without any warning, tears welled up in my eyes. 'Thanks, Mum,' I whispered to myself.

'Lovely, isn't he?' his mother said softly.

The tears were streaming down my face now. 'He's absolutely gorgeous,' I croaked.

The staff nurse came back into the room. She smiled at me. 'Go all right?' she enquired.

I nodded quietly. I was choked with emotion. I bit my bottom lip as I helped her cut the umbilical cord. She handed the baby to his mum who gave him a big kiss on the forehead.

'Here, luv,' she said and handed the baby to me. 'Give him a hug for luck.'

I looked at the pink baby and gazed down into his big blue eyes. They seemed to probe deeply into my brain. I was afraid that if I hugged him any tighter I would suffocate him.

'God bless, little one,' I whispered. 'Welcome to the world.'

'What's your name?' the patient asked me.

I told her when I had finished wiping my eyes and blowing my nose.

'Well, John it is then. His name is John. Is that all right with you?'

I was gobsmacked. 'Of course, of course,' I said. 'Thank you very much. I am very honoured. Are you sure?'

She hugged her new baby closer and said. 'Yeah, I'm sure.'

It was only afterwards that I learned that this was a set-up to let me deliver my first baby.

I visited my new namesake every day until it was time for them to go home. I was introduced to other members of the family as the doctor who brought little John into the world. When little John and his mother were leaving, she handed me a thank you card. All it said was, With thanks and love. I lived on an emotional high for the next few weeks.

My next delivery was a private patient and the consultant was assisting at the delivery. With public patients the midwife delivered the baby. If there was any problem, the assistant master of the hospital was always available. But being private or public made little or no difference. If the patient was private and the consultant was not available, the midwife delivered the baby anyway. I was holding the patient's hand and whispering what I thought to be encouraging sounds to a lady who was fully occupied expelling a human bowling ball. This was her fourth baby, the other three were boys, and this baby was delivered very quickly.

'It's a girl!' said the consultant.

The patient gave a whoop of delight and threw her arms around my neck. I must have been standing on a wet patch on the floor. I slipped and fell on top of her. She hung on like a wrestler. I couldn't move. My face was stuck into her breasts.

'John, get off the patient,' said the consultant in a tone that really meant 'bloody student'. She let me go and apologised sweetly.

❖   ❖   ❖   ❖

Paediatrics was also a major element in the first part of our final year. The hospital I attended was on the northside of the city. We did a few weeks in children's medicine and surgery with stints in the casualty. Children's casualties are busy and not the same as adult's casualty. The sick child is accompanied not only by parents but brothers, sisters and sometimes aunts, uncles, friends, neighbours and, on one memorable occasion, the family dog. There have been only two occasions in my medical career that I have been asked to look after animals. This was one. After I had seen to the little boy who had a minor problem, he asked me if I could have a look at his dog's paw as he thought it had a thorn in it.

If it made the kid happy, why not? I thought to myself.

I made sure the casualty officer wasn't around and heaved the dog up on the table. Sure enough he had a small thorn in his paw. I cleaned his paw with antiseptic and gently removed the thorn with a tweezers. The little patient was thrilled and hopped out of the office with the dog in tow. One of the staff nurses walked by with a puzzled look on her face.

'Did you have a dog in there?' she asked me.

'That's an awful thing to call a child,' I said and walked quickly down the corridor.

On a good day bedlam ruled. My first weekend on call

taught me never to use medical terminology with kids. A small boy brought in by his mother presented with a pain in his abdomen. I examined him before the casualty officer came into the cubicle.

'When was the last time you had a motion?' I asked.

'A what?' he asked.

'A motion. The last time you defecated?'

His mother pushed herself between me and the boy.

'You stop cursing at me son, you old shite!' She picked him up and backed into the corner ready for a fight.

The light dawned on me. 'I only asked him when was the last time he did a pooh!'

'Oh, you mean the last time he did a thunder in the bucket.' She held him at arm's length and shouted at him. 'Tell the doctor the last time you did a thunder?'

The child nodded in understanding and told me. Not only *when* but *what colour*.

That first weekend was a revelation to me. Kids were not just small adults with an illness, they had other problems too. Many of the parents appeared to have problems as well. During a lull we were about to go for a cup of tea when a big, worried man came into the casualty.

'My niece! My niece! She's having a fit in the car!' He caught hold of the first white-coated person he found and pulled me to his van.

'She's in the back. She's an epidemic.'

'An epidemic of what?' I asked, worried at the possible answer. There was a small breakout of lice and nits in the area. I opened the back door of the van and saw a young girl on the floor having a convulsion. She was frothing at the mouth and her body was twitching in an epileptic attack. The casualty officer climbed into the van and gave her a shot of Valium. Within a short time the attack was over. We moved her out of the van into the treatment room. Her uncle calmed down and he was asked about her history

'She has been an epidemic for a few months,' he told us. 'I think she has developed a little bit of celebrate palsy.'

The casualty officer was well used to confronting hysterical relatives.

'Well, we'll look after her for a few hours and then send her home,' he coughed politely. 'I think she is an *epileptic*,' he said the word slowly, 'and she has just had a fit.'

'Her mother will have a fit herself when she finds out. She's. in prison for the last six weeks.'

We never did get to the bottom of the 'celebrate palsy' question.

Another little girl gave me an inkling as to what her mother did as a job. I had finished putting a few sutures into her knee and was lifting her down from the stretcher. Her mother said thank you, and stood up to go.

'She needs to be seen in about six days to take the stitches out,' I reminded her. The little girl looked up at me with big brown eyes.

'Aren't you going to give my mummy a kiss goodbye?' she asked sweetly.

'I don't think that's the right thing to do,' I said.

'But all the men give mummy a kiss goodbye,' she whispered. 'And give her money as well.'

I grimaced. Her mother said nothing. I just smiled stupidly at her and nodded my head in understanding. Our learned tutors had never given us an answer for this type of problem.

❖　❖　❖　❖

There was one ward in the hospital I dreaded going into: the cancer ward. These children were tough and resilient, and could knock the breath out of you with a few words. One day I was taking blood from a child with bone cancer. She watched me like a hawk and didn't move a muscle when I stuck the needle into a tiny vein. When I took the needle out she automatically bent her arm up to stop the vein bleeding.

'How old are you?' she asked me. I told her as I squirted the blood into its container.

'I'm only seven,' she continued, 'but I think I'll be in heaven before I'm old like you.'

I could not turn around to face her. I busied myself with some bottles on the tray, holding back the tears. I wanted to get out of the cubicle as fast as I could. I gritted my teeth and made for the door, still with my back to her.

'Will you come back tomorrow?' the little voice said behind me.

I mumbled, 'Of course,' and left. To my eternal shame I didn't return.

❖   ❖   ❖   ❖

There was another part of the hospital where babies with major congenital deformities were looked after until they died. Most of these babies had horrendous nervous system defects. The little patients were kept as comfortable as humanly possible, but there was no active management to repair their defects or improve their prognoses. The consultant in surgery who looked after these little people was a very soft-hearted but practical man. He spent many hours patiently explaining to students the difference between passive and active euthanasia. Underneath all that the consultant said lay the threat that if anybody in his hospital was thought to have been a participant in active euthanasia, he would be shown just how powerful a senior consultant could really be.

I can't explain why but I had no difficulty with these hopeless cases and returned many times to the ward as a student, whereas I cringed when I passed the ward where the cancer patients were.

❖   ❖   ❖   ❖

The paediatric exams in Final Medicine finally caught up with myself and my reading room pals in December. We had little difficulty with the exams and all passed. We had only three more to go but these three – Medicine, Surgery and Ob/Gyn – were the most important exams of our career.

At this stage in our training we were learning how to shut off medicine once we left the hospital compound. One moment you might be emotionally devastated by the death of a young patient, the next you were in the local pub knocking back pints. Whether it was our way of blocking out the reality of what we had been exposed to, or whether we were a pack of alcoholics, was never discussed. We were gearing up for the awesome responsibilities that would be thrust upon us in a matter of weeks. We had been taught by some of the best teachers in medicine about the nature of disease but there was one huge chunk missing from our curriculum: we had not been taught about the patients. On reflection, I think perhaps medical students can't be taught about patients. They can learn about the diseases and the way they affect people but learning about people is a life-long process and few doctors will say they have finally got it right. My father was in practice for more than forty years and was still on the learning curve when he retired.

December of that year was one long booze-up. There were twenty-one nights of debauchery, not including Christmas. At the end of the year there was a party near Limerick. One of the nursing beauties had made the mistake of inviting some of the reading room nasties to her party. Secretly, I'm sure she hoped none of us would be daft enough to drive from Dublin and it must have gladdened her heart when it started to snow on New Year's Eve. But that didn't stop us. We drove down in my mother's Renault 4 (she still has it and has promised to leave it to me in her will) and booked into one of the local hotels. I never noticed that I was the only one of my friends to give my real name to the registration clerk in the hotel.

The party was in one of the better-off areas of Limerick. The nurse's father opened the door and eyed us with suspicion. I had on a shirt, tie and sensible jacket, but one of the others looked like a tramp. We were identified by the daughter and allowed in. I made for the bar. Free beer is a wonderful thing. You become mellower, the girls get prettier, even those who in today's politically correct times are cosmetically challenged. The New Year was ushered in. Anything in a skirt was kissed as often as possible. Any female who clung on longer than the allotted New Year's kiss demanded was a target – and I have to stress that this was a two-way street. The hostess and I made a handsome couple. We went to the front room for a cuddle and were trying to exchange clothes when her dad decided that he and I should become better acquainted. The tramp (my friend, not his daughter) and I were flung out, me because I had acted improperly with his daughter, the tramp because he was showing a group of nurses how easy it was to regurgitate the beer he had consumed out a window. It is not one of the nights that ranks high in my memory.

When I went downstairs in the hotel the next morning to pay my bill, the manageress asked if I was paying for the other 'two gentlemen' who had left earlier. They had done a runner. No wonder they had given false names.

She looked at my name and said, 'Your father looked after my father, years ago, in the Hospice in Harold's Cross.'

I nearly cried. We had a name that was well-known in medicine because of my father's work. I forked out what was owed but she knew that the other two had done a bunk. I decided to try to defuse the situation and asked her what her name was. She told me.

'My dad is still with the hospice,' I said, 'your name rings a bell. I occasionally do rounds with my father. I think I met your father recently. Fine man he is.'

'He died seven years ago,' she said flatly.

I picked up my bags, made myself as small as possible and left. The others were waiting by the car. It took me the journey back to Dublin to persuade them to pay me what they owed.

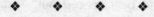

We now had six months to the final exams. All of us in the reading room were scattered around the various hospitals but looked upon the reading room as base. At least once a week we would end up in the reading room by chance or design. One night we decided to take a democratic vote: either we would study for the next six months (rejected), or we would study now and again, chase members of the opposite sex, drink copiously and study hard for the six weeks before the exams – as long as there were no parties (adopted with great enthusiasm). Looking back, perhaps we got a little out of hand.

I was alternating between a maternity hospital and St Vincent's Hospital. I was doing deliveries but I enjoyed surgery more. There was little call for obstetricians in South County Dublin as the vast majority of mothers elected to have their babies in the hospital. This is even more true today when a doctor's insurance premium for doing home deliveries has gone through the roof. Few GPs could actually afford to do home deliveries.

I did Pap smears so often I could do them with my eyes closed. I made a bet with myself once actually to try this. My patient was a little upset when she looked down and saw the doctor with his eyes closed searching around for the speculum to examine her. I think she was also surprised when the speculum headed in the wrong direction.

'Hey you! What are you doing?' she asked in a loud voice. 'Are you afraid of it or what?'

'It is part of the learning process,' I said. 'We have to be able to do examinations in the dark.'

I thought I had got away with it until she was leaving the crowded out-patients. She whispered to a few of the other patients waiting to be checked out. The next five women asked the consultant if the light could be turned off so that the young doctor could examine them in the dark. He was totally perplexed.

❖   ❖   ❖   ❖

We students had to get as much time as possible with patients before our exams so we went around the wards looking for patients with unusual problems. Some patients were, frankly, hostile. Others had such interesting illnesses that every student in the hospital would ask to examine them. One fellow had a genital problem and let it be known that only female students were welcome to examine him, gloves an optional extra.

We heard that a patient with a stroke had a problem called speech aphasia. The effects of this vary. This particular patient thought he was saying one thing while he was actually saying something else. Anything to do with strokes or cerebral vascular accidents was manna from heaven for students as these problems often came up in the final exam.

Myself and one of my colleagues from the reading room decided to see this patient. We asked the ward sister for permission to examine 'her' patient and approached him. He was sitting up in bed, no drips or monitors around him. He looked as if he was on a holiday. He nodded and smiled when we introduced ourselves. He had a little bit of difficulty trying to shake our hands but otherwise seemed healthy. I sat on the bed, folded my arms and in a serious manner started my interrogation.

'What happened a few days ago that brought you into the hospital?' I asked innocently.

He looked as if he was going to answer with no problem. He beamed and said, 'A carthorse,' he paused, 'full of cowshit on the main road.'

What a funny way to have an accident, I thought to myself. 'You were hit by a carthorse carrying a load of cowshi–, er, manure on a main road?' I asked.

'Yes, yes, and the mouse vanished up into his own little hole!'

My fellow student started to giggle and I knew that if I moved my head so much as an inch I would start giggling too. Although the patient couldn't respond to our questions he understood what was going on. After a few more questions my serious demeanour cracked and I started to smirk. It was like starting to laugh at a funeral; no matter what you do you cannot stop. Unfortunately it was visiting time and his family were outside the cubicle listening to the whole thing. They were a little unhappy. Another lesson learnt that day: do not examine patients during visiting hours.

❖　　❖　　❖　　❖

Six weeks before the exams we began to prepare in earnest. Parties and booze-ups were put on the back-burner. We rationed them to only three a week – a major scale-down. There was a disco near the hospital and one Friday night I went there for a bit of relaxation with some friends. We seldom met any girls, we went for a few drinks, a laugh and then home after a brief excursion to one of the clubs in Leeson Street. I was minding my own business when I noticed a very slim blonde walking by me. I seldom asked anyone to dance but this woman was different.

'Excuse me,' I said. 'Would you care to dance?'

She turned around to me and smiled. 'Not right now, thank you,' she said with a look that said, get lost.

'Why not?' I asked.

She didn't expect that. 'Because I have a drink in one hand, a cigarette in the other, and I'm holding my handbag under my arm.'

My mind was racing. I could not let this one get off the hook so easily.

'OK, I'll hold your handbag, buy you another drink and you can have a cigarette afterwards.'

'No, I still don't want to dance but I will talk to you if you like,' she said sweetly.

I gulped. 'Talk to me, talk to me? I didn't come here for a bloody English lesson.' How could I have known that we would be married within two years?

She finally told me two very important details: her name was Joan and she had nothing to do with nursing. I dropped her home, but a proper relationship was not to start until a few months later.

❖ ❖ ❖ ❖

We were getting into our stride now with the study. We tried very hard to limit outings to the agreed three a week, but it just wasn't possible and we had to bow to the inevitable. Perhaps subconsciously we knew that our wayward lifestyle was coming to an end and that with luck we would start work as interns on the first of July. We were in a frenzy of activity both inside and outside the hospital. It was a rare night that we didn't finish up in the Ballsbridge Inn. If there was no action there the Merrion Inn was a reliable back up. We didn't notice the weeks passing.

The senior lecturer in the hospital posted our continuous assessment results. We had done better than we expected. I got a mark which was good enough to secure a job in the hospital if I passed my finals. I began to think about what I would like to do as an intern. There was a rotation for six months in General and Plastic Surgery and a small involvement in Ophthalmic Surgery that looked interesting. I also wanted to do Cardiology and General Medicine.

One of the more flamboyant general surgeons, James Murphy, had his out-patients clinic on Fridays. I went to see him.

'I was wondering if I could be your intern for the next six months,' I asked, my heart in my mouth. He had given us a rough time as students in his clinics and lectures.

He stood on the weighing scales just inside the out-patients door. 'You're mad, wanting to work for me. Tell you what, if you weigh more than me you can have the job.'

Kind of an odd qualification to have, I thought. I stood on the scales. I was twelve pounds heavier.

'OK,' he said, 'first of July, my intern. Don't be late.'

I had my job. Now only the minor problem of the finals stood in the way.

❖   ❖   ❖   ❖

Things started to hot up and we did mock finals with whoever would spare the time. It was during this time that I came across two doctors who were definitely odd. We were in the habit of asking students in other hospitals whether they had patients with interesting illnesses so we could go and examine them. This was important as most of the St Vincent's students would have their final examination in different hospitals around the city. Anybody with a medical curiosity could be on for the finals. I locked on to a doctor in one of the other hospitals and we did some ward rounds. On one round a staff nurse told this doctor that one of the male patients needed his urinary catheter changed – this is a small rubber tube inserted through the penis into the bladder. The catheter is passed through the penis into the bladder and a small balloon at its tip is inflated to keep it in place and stop it leaking. This little balloon, holding about 10cc of sterile water, has to be deflated before removal for obvious reasons.

No matter what he did this doctor couldn't deflate the balloon. The patient was about eighty years old and had had his prostate gland operated on. After a few minutes the doctor cursed loudly and tugged hard on the catheter. A howl of surprise issued from the patient. My eyes popped wide open when I realised what had happened – the catheter had been removed without being deflated.

'Now,' said the doctor, 'no more operations on your prostate, old man.' He walked off.

The staff nurse was rooted to the spot, her jaw halfway to the floor. She had never seen this procedure before. The patient's penis looked as if it had been rebored with a drainpipe. Luckily he appeared to suffer no permanent problems.

The other unorthodox doctor worked in a hospital I visited only once as a student. He hated getting out of bed, even if he was on call. A patient arrived early one Sunday morning. With great reluctance, the nurses woke up the doctor. His mood was not improved when he heard that the patient had a dose of the runs, a problem seldom encountered in hospital. However he was very polite and asked the patient to lie on his stomach and pulled down his pants as he wanted to examine him rectally. The doctor placed one paddle of the defibrillator on each of the patient's buttocks and defibbed his arse. The patient let out a yodel, his bowels seemed to explode and he disappeared out the door. The doctor replaced the paddles of the defibrillator on the stand.

'There,' he said. 'That scared the shit out of him.'

He mused briefly about writing to one of the medical journals about his new novel way of treating diarrhoea and went back off to bed.

Chapter 7

The Finals

We had the papers in Obstetrics and Gynaecology first. Our revision for the past few weeks saved us. The week before the exam my friends and I were doing fourteen to fifteen hours of study a day with few or no clinics. The parties were forgotten, the ladies put on hold. After larking about for a considerable number of years we had to take things very seriously. The papers in Ob/Gyn would be fairly easy as would those in Surgery and Medicine. Then we'd have a week to wait for the clinics and orals. If you had done a poor paper you could always drag yourself up with good marks in these. We put in a sixteen-hour day studying before our final clinic examination in Ob/Gyn in the National Maternity Hospital.

The exam started at nine in the morning and we had to wait our turn in the hospital library. I hoped to get an obstetrics case and not a gynaecological case. In obstetrics you could only get a woman who was pregnant or who had just had her baby. A gynae patient could have anything wrong with 'the works'.

I was called out and introduced to a lady who had just had a baby. Saved, I thought. She was an 'ordinary' post natal case. No complications, easy to examine and very relaxed. When I finished the history and examination I asked her if there was anything I should know. There wasn't, she said, and we had a chat about holidays and her kids while I waited for the consultants to question me.

All went well and I felt I had a chance of an honour, but my chances were dashed at the oral examination. I got some words hopelessly mixed up: multiparous, meaning having more than one baby, and nulliparous, meaning no pregnancies. The examiners laughed out loud when I used the word 'nutiperous'. I didn't get my honour.

The following morning we had our Surgery Clinic in a hospital which is now closed, Sir Patrick Dunne's. My patient was a thin, wizened old man. He appeared to be enjoying the limelight. I shook his hand and sat on the bed.

'What appears to be the problem?' I probed, putting on my stethoscope.

'I've got the scutters,' he said in a thin high voice.

I froze. 'The *what*?'

'The scutters. I've had them for about six weeks.'

What on earth were the scutters? my brain screamed. 'The scutters?' I asked hoarsely. 'Could you explain that?'

'You know the shits. Black shits, like feckin' tar.'

I let out a breath of air. He had melena, a serious condition which indicated bleeding in the stomach. He was thin, looked a little pale and jaundiced, and had a large lymph gland in his left neck called a Verchov's node. His liver felt a little knobbly. He had lost his appetite and felt very weak. I diagnosed cancer of the stomach which had spread to his liver. His prognosis to my mind was hopeless. His GP had told him he had a stomach ulcer that was going bad and he had been admitted into hospital three days before the exam. He had counted the number of students and junior doctors who had examined him before and during the exam. I was the twenty-second. I had little doubt that they all came to the same unpleasant conclusion.

The examining surgeons came into the cubicle and asked me about the patient. I went through my findings but did not give my diagnosis until we stepped out into the hall.

'Well?' one of them asked.

'Stomach cancer with metathesis in the liver,' I replied.

He nodded. 'Treatment?'

'His cancer is so advanced, only supportive care. No indications for surgery.'

'Poor devil,' whispered the other surgeon.

They took me to the 'minors' room where there were less frightening cases to chat about – a case of varicose veins, an infected sebaceous cyst, a lump behind a patient's knee that I diagnosed as a Baker's cyst.

'Do well in the orals this afternoon and you should get your honour,' said the surgeon.

My future boss, James Murphy, was one of the two examiners that afternoon. I sat in front of the desk and waited. The Professor of Surgery told me he was going to show me x-rays of the abdomen. He would ask if the x-rays were of the upper or lower bowel and what I thought was wrong. He put one of the x-rays on the viewer.

'Now, John, this is a barium study of the bowel. Is it upper or lower intestine?'

'Upper bowel,' I said nervously.

'Very good. Now, what pathology do you see in this x-ray?'

The only thing that a student could possibly be shown would be a cancer of the stomach, an ulcer in the stomach or an ulcer in the duodenum. I peered at the x-ray and decided on the stomach cancer. The professor nodded with approval and showed me another x-ray.

'Lower intestine,' I said.

'Very good,' said the professor. He showed me another picture.

'Also the lower intestine,' I said.

'Excellent, John. Now what do you think of this?'

And so it went on for fifteen minutes. When the little bell sounded time up, the professor turned towards his companion and had a brief chat.

They both smiled at me. 'We think you deserve an honour.'

One pass, one honour.

The exam in Medicine was the following day. That night I was flicking through a few books in the reading room when a few of the others came in. They had all done well in Surgery, except for one student who felt he had failed. Somebody mentioned a pint and off we went to the Ballsbridge Inn, where a pint turned into numerous pints. We forgot that the following day was one of the biggest exams of our lives. I crawled into bed about two o'clock and the next day was waiting to be called for the clinical examination with a slight headache. I popped two mints into my mouth to disguise the alcohol halitosis that I suspected could kill my patient.

The patient sat on the bed, his arms folded, waiting to be questioned. I introduced myself and asked him why he had been admitted.

'Dizzy spells.'

Dizzy spells are not one of the student's favourites. They could mean anything from bowels to brains. You could spend hours examining a dizzy patient and still be no wiser. If the examiners took an instant dislike to you (and bloodshot eyes and horrible breath tended to encourage that), they could easily shoot you down on cases like this. The patient looked as comfortable as if he had seen it all before. I took a chance.

'And what else is wrong with you?'

'I've got cirrhosis of the liver,' he said in a low voice.

I punched the air and whispered, 'Yes! yes! yes!'

'I've been in three years in a row with cirrhosis,' he

99

whispered in a conspiratorial kind of way. 'Funny how it always seems to be around exam time for the young doctors.'

'Why are you in with dizzy spells then?'

He shrugged his shoulders. 'I don't know. I suppose it's something to do with the cirrhosis.'

'OK,' I said, 'when the examiners come in I'll tell them that you were admitted with a liver problem. Would that be OK?'

He nodded. 'Sure, Doc.'

He was a professional patient. He was easy to examine. He knew all about his liver disease and the signs one should look for. The examiners came in and stood at the foot of the bed.

'I see this patient was admitted for investigation of dizzy spells among other things,' one of them said. He held the clipboard tight to his chest as if I was trying to take a peek at it.

'No, sir. He was admitted with a liver problem according to himself.' I looked at the patient. He nodded with great solemnity.

The professor searched frantically through his clipboard for the notes to this patient. 'It says "patient with dizzy spells" here,' he muttered to himself. 'All right, tell us about the cirrhosis.'

I took a deep breath and started my presentation, pointing out the various signs that the illness had produced. Dizzy spells were not mentioned. My time was up. I shook the patient's hand and whispered my thanks.

My second patient was a thin woman with emphysema. She had the classic signs and symptoms of advanced lung disease from nicotine-stained fingers to laboured breathing. She spoke very little throughout the exam and looked exhausted at the end. When the examiners came in they took one look at her and decided to take her off their list. I heard that she died a few days later.

The results were to be read out the next day in Belfield campus. I told my parents that the results were to be read out the day after that – if I failed it would give me twenty-four hours to leave the country. I could, of course, repeat, but I had done enough repeating in my earlier medical years.

❖　　❖　　❖　　❖

The whole class gathered in one of the theatres in Belfield. All of us from the reading room sat in a row, chatting nervously while we waited for the results. We had entered the theatre as students, we hoped to leave as doctors.

The administrator walked in with a huge black book and put it on the desk in front of him.

Judgement day had arrived!

'Here are the results of the final medical examination. The names will be read in alphabetical order and after each name a pass or reject will be indicated.'

Reject! What a terrible word to tell somebody they had failed their exam. I was shaking with nerves, my mouth was dry, I was dying to go to the toilet. The administrator started his litany. After each result there would be a whoop of delight or an awkward silence as somebody was rejected. Time seemed to stop when he came to my name.

'John Fleetwood. Pass.'

I exploded with relief. I gave a loud 'Yeeees!' and put my head on the bench in front of me muttering, 'Thank you, God, thank you, thank you, thank you.'

All along the row there were yells of delight as our names were called out. Until the very last name was called.

'Reject'.

One of our reading room gang had failed. A very popular

student had had a terrible surgical final. He had known before the result that he had little chance. He just shook his head.

It was all over. I was a doctor. I felt ten feet tall. Outside the theatre we danced around and hugged each other, some crying, most laughing, the stress of the past years wiped out with one word: pass. I commiserated to the best of my lightheaded ability with those who had to spend another six months as students.

❖   ❖   ❖   ❖

The party that night was one of those bitter-sweet affairs. We started some time in the early evening and by a miracle made it safely to the Ballsbridge Inn. When I opened the door of the pub I was greeted by one of the quieter class members, naked except for a pair of frilly knickers. The girl I was with thought he looked very nice and broke off our relationship soon afterwards. The night ended at a party close to where my parents lived. Fortunately I had left the car at home and we all tried hard to identify with my Finals patient with cirrhosis.

We had the month of June off before we started as interns. I decided to buy a second-hand sports car and spend a few weeks fixing it up. During that time everything that resembled the fair sex was fair game and I went out with a considerable number of young women. I also went out with my future wife, Joan. Although I had promised myself that I would not get involved with a woman during my intern year, I started going out with Joan on the fifth of July, five days after I started my professional career. We became engaged (unofficially) after six weeks.

It sneaks up on you, doesn't it?

Chapter 8

Intern

*A*lthough I had three degrees, MB, BCH, BAO, after my name they did nothing to help me with my very first ward round. I arrived on the ward at half-seven in the morning, met the senior houseman, the registrar, and my intern partner, Con Cronin. Con and I had to get to know our new patients before our consultant appeared so we could present the patients to him. We were halfway through our familiarisation when the consultant appeared on the ward. We had started on one end of the ward, he started at the other end where the patients were strangers to us. I think he did it on purpose.

An old saying in medicine is that a patient should never have themselves admitted to a hospital on the first of July if they can help it. In the old days at least, new interns coming on often had scarcely a clue. The morbidity and the mortality rate seemed to us to edge up for the first few weeks while we came to grips with new responsibilities.

On our very first day as doctors, Con and I were on call all night. We admitted patient after patient to the surgical service, everything from road traffic accidents to acute pancreatitis. At about three in the morning I was heavy with importance and fatigue. I was called to a male patient who was in a considerable amount of pain after an operation. I checked his chart to see if he had any allergies and decided to give him an intravenous injection of a powerful painkiller. The sister on the ward was a little dubious and suggested that an intra-muscular injection would be safer.

I'm the doctor, I thought. I decide what to give and how to give it.

The patient, a nice man, had an acute allergic reaction and we spent a frantic fifteen minutes reviving him.

It was an unpleasant lesson to learn. When the ward sister 'suggested' something, I decided, it was generally a good idea to follow her advice. This patient, however, was thrilled to have a new doctor looking in on him every thirty minutes or so. He was not at all surprised when I examined him from head to foot each time.

At eight the next morning with about two hours' sleep behind us, Con and I presented ourselves in the operating theatre. Only one intern was needed for surgery, we were told, and as Con had no great desire to be a surgeon he volunteered to stay on the ward.

Our first case was a patient with a gall bladder and I scrubbed with James Murphy. We were joined by two students and we launched into the patient's abdomen with great zeal. All went well until the end. Mr Murphy had inserted a tube called a T-tube into the patient's bile duct so that the bile could drain and be observed for a few days. The tube was brought out from the bile duct up through the layers of muscle and out through the skin. As we were sewing up the abdomen, one of the students removed a retractor, an instrument that helps the surgeon see into the operating site, with too much gusto. The T-tube came out as well like a little tail flopping about on the end of the retractor.

'I don't believe it,' stammered Mr Murphy. 'In all my years as a surgeon I have never seen that before. What's your name, eejit?'

The student was frozen with fright. It may have been my second day as an intern but it was his first time assisting at an operation. I could see his mouth working frantically underneath his mask. From beneath his gown he made a sound suspiciously like a fart.

'Well?' demanded Mr Murphy. For one horrible moment I thought the student was going to move his bowels.

'Eamon,' he gulped. He held the retractor like a weapon.

'Eamon, Eamon,' sighed Mr Murphy. 'Do you know what happens to a student who whips out a T-tube?'

Eamon shook his head violently from side to side, his cheeks making a sloppy noise.

Mr Murphy continued, 'He has to buy me ten cigars.'

'Huh?' Eamon swallowed.

'When the shop opens across the road you can run over and buy me ten cigars.'

When the operation was finished Eamon went off on his errand. He didn't bother to look behind him at the windows of the operating room, so he didn't see us all roaring laughing.

We finished in the OR late that Saturday afternoon and went down for a post-op ward round. I had a bite to eat and thought that I deserved a few pints in the Ballsbridge Inn.

The pub was very quiet that night as the other new doctors from the hospital and I were all wrecked. We sipped our pints and exchanged stories. It comforted me to find out that I wasn't the only one who had an awful lot to learn.

On Monday morning I returned to the operating room for the list in plastic surgery and I was in the theatre until four o'clock. Then ward rounds again until around six. For the next six months I was in the operating theatre four days a week, on duty at least every Friday night and working one weekend – from Friday morning to Monday evening – in five. The normal working week averaged out at between eighty-five and ninety-five hours depending on your enthusiasm. A slow week was when the consultant went on holiday and we did a leisurely sixty hours. You could stay in the ward all day and all night if you wanted to. In reality interns stayed until the day's work was finished, no matter how long that took. It was just part of the job and we knew it would last only one long energy-sapping year. Nowadays things may have improved slightly, but not much.

Our general surgical patients ranged from the minor – lumps and bumps – to the major – breast cancer and intestinal problems. We did the hard cases first when we were fresh and kept the easier ones for later in the afternoon.

One Thursday we had to operate on two patients who had similar problems. They had a condition called Crohn's disease where part of the intestine becomes so inflamed it has to be removed. Mr Murphy and I removed part of the intestine of one patient, while the registrar, Paul, and SHO, Alex, were in the adjoining theatre removing part of the intestines of the other patient. Both operations ended after about three hours. Both patients had colostomies, little bags attached to the skin where the intestine was brought out to the skin surface. Colostomy bags collect the bowel motions, as the patient more often than not has had his rectum removed as well. There were no complications and both patients were brought back to the ward for post-op care.

One of the patients, George, was awake and talking in a very short time. He accepted the colostomy bag with little or no comment, knowing that he would have it for the rest of his life. He was only worried that he could not have a puff on his pipe. Within two days he was up and about, walking down the corridors with a little help from the two nurses. They turned a blind eye whenever George had a quick smoke – out of the sight of the staff nurse of course. The other patient didn't do so well. He couldn't come to terms with the bag. While George was getting better the other man appeared to lose hope. Physically he was in good shape but every time we examined him, he looked down at the bag and mumbled that 'he wasn't all there'.

One night before I went off on a date with Joan, George called me over to his bed.

'That fella has no bottle, Doc,' he said, his ever-present unlit pipe in his mouth.

I asked him exactly what he meant.

'He's not going to make it,' he said matter-of-factly.

'He's doing fine, George,' I whispered. 'He'll be up and out in no time.'

'Out maybe, but not walking. In a box.'

I looked over at the other patient and felt a chill in my spine. I left the ward with an uneasy feeling that perhaps George was right in his assessment. The patient with no 'bottle' died that night. He developed a clot in his leg which travelled to his lung and killed him. George on the other hand, took the whole thing in his stride and left the hospital two weeks later. Mr Murphy did not take kindly to a death under his care and was rightly upset.

Mr Murphy decided to let Paul, the registrar, do all the gall bladders and that I would assist. Every day in surgery we would do gall bladders – in total I must have assisted Paul in about twenty in the six months I was with them.

Between operations we would have a cup of coffee while the next patient was prepared for the knife. Paul had numerous friends who were policemen and regaled us with stories about the goings on of the law. He liked ballads and among his many songs was, 'Me Granny Drowned in the Pool at Lourdes'. When Pope John Paul came to Dublin I renamed this ballad 'Me Granny was Killed by the Pope-Mobile in

1979'. But, although we worked together for six months, I never really got to know Paul. He was a bit of an enigma and disappeared from the scene a few years later. I last heard that he was working somewhere in the Middle East. Alex, the senior house officer, had the unusual distinction of having his Fellowship in surgery before he was a registrar. He was a real gentleman and in our six months I never saw him get annoyed or frustrated with any of the interns. Both of us had sports cars but there the similarity ended. He would never stoop to the low art of 'slagging' people, especially to their faces.

I, however, learned how to slag in the reading room where one could be reduced to tears of laughter by a good opponent. At happy hour in various pubs, we let off steam. It was our unwritten rule that you could say anything to anyone and no offence could be inferred or taken. Strangers could not understand the verbal barbs that were exchanged between so-called friends. You had to be very quick to get in the last jab or humiliation was the order of the day.

❖　❖　❖　❖

I was also working with the plastic surgeon, Séamus O Riain, who went to great pains to show me his craft. He allowed me to do some minor surgery because the registrar of plastic surgery was also working with another team. I saw my first face lift and was astonished at the amount of reshaping that had to be done. When I assisted him at fixing up an accident victim, I saw the true expertise of a plastic surgeon. The majority of our work was on accident victims.

Learning the art of medicine involved the occasional surprise. One Sunday I was in the ward admitting 'plastics' patients when the ward sister told me that a new patient had arrived. I pulled back the curtains and faced a gift from the gods. She was eighteen years old and had come in to have her breasts reduced.

'My boobs are too big,' she said.

I thought they looked wonderful. The fact that she was going to allow surgery on them seemed like a crime to me. I excused myself and went out to the ward sister, a nun who was what all nuns should be, wonderful. She used to bring the hungover interns and students into her room and give them shots of Maxalon so they wouldn't get sick. She was the type of nun junior doctors prayed for when they came on to the wards.

'That girl wants her breasts reduced,' I said. 'I think she's daft.'

'Have you asked her why?'

In my shock I hadn't.

'Go back and talk to her about the problem an eighteen-year-old girl with big breasts has.'

'But they're perfect,' I said.

'To you maybe, but not to her. Off you go.'

I went back to the young lady and learned about the unpleasant side of having big breasts – premenstrual tenderness, taunts from the boys who called her 'thunder-tits', the embarrassment of hiding your own body.

I assisted Séamus O Riain the next morning and marvelled at the way he made her breasts more presentable for her. A few days later when she examined herself she was thrilled. She had been reduced from a size 38 to a size 34 and left the hospital with a little less bounce than when she had entered.

❖   ❖   ❖   ❖

James Murphy had a wicked humour on occasion. This was usually directed at me. I asked him once if he would look after a friend of mine who had an early duodenal ulcer.

'He wanted the best,' I said.

Mr Murphy beamed.

'But the best wasn't available, so I suggested you,' I added jokingly.

But he got his own back on me. From then on I was given jobs and duties that were unappetising to say the least. We had done a total colectomy, that is removed the whole of the large bowel, and Mr Murphy told me to bring the removed organ into the sluice room and to open it lengthwise. The smell nearly made me vomit. I could feel the bile rising in my throat as I slipped the scissors along its whole length. A senior houseman came in and asked me what I was doing.

'Opening the colon,' I said, gagging.

'The pathologists usually do that,' he said casually. 'Never seen an intern do it before. Smelly, isn't it?'

I felt like twisting the intestine around his neck. It was in the same sluice room that one of my fellow interns lost a lung. A patient with lung cancer had his lung removed and the consultant asked the intern to take the lung into the sluice room and wash it. The sluice had a one-way suction machine that sucked down any bits of blood or discarded tissue into some unnamed hell in the bowels of the hospital. While the intern was cleaning the lung it slipped from his hands and was gobbled up by the machine. His explanations to the surgeon, according to those present, were gibberish.

Near the end of my surgical internship I assisted at the longest operation I ever attended. It lasted eleven-and-a-half hours. We used microscopes to reconstruct a nerve in a patient's arm. He had broken the arm some months before and when it was reset one of the nerves was found to be actually within the healed fracture. The nerve had died and we had to rejoin the two ends with a nerve from his ankle. We started at ten in the morning and finished at half-past nine that evening. The surgeon and I only left the theatre on two occasions to have a pee. We rescrubbed and went back to work. Afterwards, I went into the Ballsbridge Inn without showering, for a few pints. My fellow drinkers mumbled that I looked terrible and smelt worse.

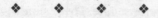

In November Joan and myself decided it was time to get officially engaged. Being a romantic at heart I thought that it was right and proper to ask her dad for her hand in marriage and he gave his permission and blessings.

My family greeted the news with whoops of joy. They had finally got rid of me!

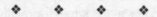

I was called one night to see a patient who had had a major operation three weeks before. Lying on the stretcher was a thin old man surrounded by a gang of students. He was on a drip and his abdomen was covered with a sterile gown.

'His intestines have popped out,' said the casualty officer.

'Oh, yes?' I queried. I was somewhat startled. I asked the patient, who did not seem to be in any distress, what had happened.

'I was in me bed with me wife and I coughed. I could feel something burst down in me belly. Me sausages had come out.'

I lifted the sterile dressing and resting on his abdomen was a considerable portion of his innards.

111

A senior registrar popped in to have a look. 'OK, bring him upstairs and we'll shove them back in again,' was all he said. We brought the old man up to the operating room, repaired the damage and he left the hospital ten days later, no worse for wear.

On Friday afternoons we had our out-patients clinic. About forty people would be given an appointment for two o'clock and would then have to wait hours to be seen by the surgeon. To this day I have yet to figure out why all the patients were given the same appointment time. These clinics were wonderful from the teaching point of view. Mr Murphy was unusual as he had done a stint as a GP in his early days and went to some lengths to inform students of a little-known fact that GPs generally made the diagnosis before the patient was sent to him for further treatment. Hospital medicine and general practice were two different sides of the medical coin and students tended to be taught the hospital side of medicine. Many students and junior hospital doctors still look upon GPs as failed hospital doctors who could not make it into the world of real medicine and it must be said that GPs believe that hospital doctors would not have a clue how to practise family medicine.

At one of these clinics I was at my desk when an elderly gentleman sat down in front of me. He had come by bus from the country to see the surgeon. He arrived without an appointment or a letter from his GP, and, although we were full, the girl on reception took pity on him and squeezed him onto our list.

'What's the problem?' I asked.

'I can see my guts,' he said.

'Really? Where can you see them?' I enquired, wondering if the psychiatric ward was missing a patient. He pulled up his shirt and pointed to an old dirty bandage over the right side of his abdomen.

'Under here. Will you have a look?'

When we removed the bandage his intestines were quite visible. He told us that for a few weeks he had felt a discomfort over his the right side of his abdomen, especially when he rounded up the sheep on the mountain. A few days later his skin became itchy and red. He thought he had an abscess and waited for it 'to point'. It seemed to 'burst out' of him and he could see his guts inside the hole. He only got worried when, as he said, he seemed to be 'doing me motions through me side'. He wanted us to fix him up so that he could go back to the farm. It looked as if he had developed an unusual variation of a diverticular abscess which had worked its way through his abdominal wall. Needless to say, his case was unusually interesting and was presented at a surgical conference the following Wednesday. He went home, on the bus, after two weeks. I was full of admiration for him; he was one tough man.

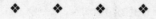

One of my colleagues from the reading room, Donal, got engaged halfway through my intern year. He decided to have a stag party in the BBI to celebrate. I was working that day and arrived at the gathering about eight o'clock. The party was only an hour old and there was a promise in the air of a wonderful night ahead. There were thirteen of us, all doctors, all professional people.

I sat beside a friend and after ordering a pint casually whispered into his ear, 'Drop your trousers.' I expected him to laugh and decline. Not only did the trousers come off but so did the rest of his clothes. It was as if a floodgate had opened. Trousers, shirts, socks, Y-fronts were flung about with a complete disregard for the other patrons in the packed pub. We had a pint glass on the table for a pool of money. We each put in ten pounds, adding up to a healthy £130 – and that was in the late seventies.

The barman came over. 'Gents, if you don't put your clothes back on there'll be no more drinks.'

Dutifully we put any clothes that were around back on, no matter whose they were, ordered the pints – and undressed again when the beer arrived. We had a Biggest Bum competition, and invited some of the hospital nurses who were backed up well away from us against the far wall to become judges. Before we got to the dangly bits, Donal was found unconscious in the toilet. Donal is a big man and it took four of us to pull him out onto the floor of the bar. He lay there, spreadeagled in all his glory. A small pyramid of cigarette butts and ice was constructed carefully around his genitals. It looked very pretty. A more senior doctor present noticed that Donal was not well and dragged him back to casualty where the many G & Ts he had consumed were pumped unceremoniously out of him.

Back at the stag party things had warmed up. Paddy, who was to become my partner, wandered into the crowd wearing nothing but a shirt sleeve. The nurses he spoke to wouldn't look below his neck. While he was off in the crowd the rest of us put our clothes back on and sat down. When there were twelve others running around the pub without clothes it was great fun, not when he suddenly found himself alone and naked. His underpants were hanging from a wall light, and pieces of his shirt had been used to wipe the table, his trousers were not to be seen. But Paddy was not embarrassed. He had a cigarette in one hand, a pint in the other and was in that wonderful state of lubrication when you don't give a damn. He wiggled his hips, called us chickens and turned back to his audience of young wide-eyed nurses.

We looked at each other, whipped off our clothes again and joined in. The following morning many junior hospital doctors were unwell – except for Donal. He had had a great night's sleep after he had been pumped out.

❖   ❖   ❖   ❖

It took a long weekend on duty to finally get me into trouble with the night matron. I was called to the neurosurgical ward to put a condom catheter on a young man who was unconscious after an accident which had damaged his brain. A condom catheter is slipped onto the patient's penis so that his urine flows into a little collecting bag. It is better for the patient and stops him wetting the bed. There were two nurses on their first night duty and they came with me to see the procedure. I took the condom catheter out of its packet and, in a moment of wickedness, put it on my nose and chased one of the nurses out of the room and into the corridor. I almost knocked over the night matron who was doing her rounds. She glared at the nurse and looked at the offending article attached to my nose.

'Interesting use of a condom catheter, Doctor,' she said.

'Yes, Matron,' I replied sheepishly. I wanted to dig a hole and disappear. The nurse was trying to melt into the wall.

But the matron sniffed and walked off with no reprimand, which worried me. The night matron reigns over the hospital. It was not wise to tangle with her.

I got back to bed about two in the morning and looked forward to a few hours of uninterrupted sleep as Con had offered to cover for me until the morning. The phone went at half-past five. I fumbled for the receiver, wondering what the emergency was.

'Yes?' I said yawning.

'This is the night matron, Doctor.'

I snapped awake instantly. 'Yes, Matron, what can I do for you?'

'I am playing Ludo in the casualty nurses' office and I need a partner.' She put the phone down.

This was my punishment. I struggled out of bed and made my way to the casualty. I played Ludo for an hour and my escapade was not mentioned once.

❖   ❖   ❖   ❖

Towards Christmas, my tonsils were at me in a big way. I decided to admit myself during my holidays under the consultant ENT (Earn, Nose and Throat) surgeon. I would become my worst nightmare, a patient. Although I was an intern in the hospital I had to be admitted by the intern on call. My fellow patients thought it hilarious that one of the hospital doctors was now a resident among them. The amusement turned to amazement when the intern arrived in a full scrub suit, holding a sigmoidoscope. I was in to get my tonsils whipped out. A sigmoidoscope is used for examining patient's rectums. Sheer fortune intervened when the matron made her rounds and wanted to know which intern had had the cheek to steal one of her beds.

The next morning I was wheeled down to the OR through my own ward. I felt very relaxed after the pre-med medication and said goodbye to everyone I met. When I awoke I felt surprisingly well, said, 'I'm okay' and dozed off again.

My few days as a patient made me a little more aware of the anxieties patients have when admitted to hospital. As a doctor, I knew what was going to happen, my fellow patients didn't. But for once they had a doctor as a patient and much of my recuperation was taken up with answering their questions.

Chapter 9

Cardiology Intern

On the first of January I started as an intern in Cardiology and General Medicine. I had requested this job some months before as, since my days as a research student, I had enjoyed Cardiology. I was also a member of the cardiac arrest team along with the registrar and SHO, two of the best doctors I ever worked with, and my fellow intern, Mary, who must have had enormous patience to put up with me. We carried arrest bleeps and when anybody in the hospital had a cardiac arrest our bleeps went off. This could happen during a meal, in the loo, on ward rounds, anytime.

On duty one night we got an arrest call to one of the surgical wards. A French sailor had had what appeared to be a cardiac arrest and all hell broke loose. Actually he had only fainted and woke up to find himself surrounded by a hoard of doctors and nurses. He spoke rapidly in French and indicated that he wanted to go to the toilet. One of the nurses produced a urinal bottle and handed it to him. He gave a gallant shrug, dropped his pyjama bottoms and sat on the bottle on the bed to move his bowels. We just stood there and watched him balancing on the bottle, muttering and grunting happily while he relieved himself.

'Bon,' he said finally, and handed the bottle back to the nurse. We left the ward happy in the knowledge that a French sailor would have some strange stories to tell about Irish medicine.

My first week on the cardiac unit was actually very quiet. Even on night duty we all got to bed and I thought if things went on like this I was in for a quiet six months. The next few weeks made up for my brief rest. I seldom got to bed and had the unusual experience of having a patient drop dead literally into my arms.

I was passing the toilets one morning and smelt cigarette smoke coming from one of the cubicles. Some of these patients, even if they were in with a heart attack, still had to have the odd puff. The door opened and a patient who had been admitted a few days earlier with a minor heart attack shuffled out, leaving a fog of smoke behind him. I had to look serious. Smoking and heart attacks were not compatible.

'John,' I asked, 'were you smoking in there?'

He didn't say anything. He just stood in front of me, his face pale.

Fright, I thought. I had to lighten up a little.

'You shouldn't smoke after you have had a heart attack. You might get another.'

He did. There and then. His eyes rolled and he fell dead into my arms. For a few seconds I was stunned. We were near the door of the cardiac unit and there was an empty bed just inside.

'Arrest, arrest,' I shouted, and dragged him into the bed and started trying to revive him. In the blink of an eye the place was full of medics. After thirty minutes we knew it was hopeless and pronounced him dead. The post mortem showed that he had ruptured his heart, a situation that is invariably fatal.

We got an arrest call one morning in the casualty. We expected an elderly patient. We didn't expect a nineteen-year-old female student. The casualty officer and registrar were working frantically on her. She had a rash like tiny blue pinpricks all over her body. The registrar said she had come in conscious with what appeared to be early meningitis. In the middle of his initial examination she had said, 'I feel terrible,' and collapsed.

We restarted her heart and decided to take her immediately to the intensive care unit. On the way she arrested again. I was doing cardiac massage while we charged down the corridors past startled patients and visitors. Unfortunately, our work was in vain and she was pronounced dead one hour later. She had died from meningococcal septicaemia, a fairly uncommon but terrible infection that overwhelms the body. It is also contagious and we had to take antibiotics as protection for a week afterwards.

Her death was the first the cardiac arrest team suffered in a run of unsuccessful resuscitations. I became a little depressed at our failures. My mood was further lowered when I admitted a forty-six-year-old with angina to the cardiac unit. She was very frightened and asked me if she was going to die.

Lightheartedly I said, 'Don't worry. You'll be here for a long time to come, that I promise.'

She arrested about an hour later and died.

I hit one of the lowest points of my life. I got a further bashing when I stayed up one night with a desperately ill patient. He arrested a number of times during the night but in the early morning I thought he had finally stabilised. I was famished and nipped down to the hospital dining-room for breakfast. When I got back to the cardiac unit the team on call were working on him again. My bleeper hadn't worked. Doctors and nurses were swarming all over him. I stood to one side and let them get on with the job. He was defibbed so many times to try and restart his heart that even the students present got the opportunity to shock him. When he was finally pronounced dead the tears welled up in my eyes. The next few days were as if a fog was clouding my mind. I did what was necessary to ensure the patients' welfare but my heart, excuse the pun, was very heavy.

But things started to improve and as the cardiac unit started to save lives and pulled people back from the brink my spirits rose. I enjoyed getting to the unit in the early morning to examine the patients who had arrived overnight. I learned that panicking at arrests was not in the patients' interest and the unit became a smooth-working arrest team.

I also learned that accidentally switching off pacemakers caused a patient unnecessary discomfort!

We were in the hospital x-ray department one night putting in an external pacemaker to a lady whose heart just wouldn't beat fast enough to keep her conscious. We finally manoeuvred the pacemaker wire into the right ventricle and turned on the machine. The patient was awake within seconds and looking around her. The registrar asked me to fine-tune the pacemaker. By mistake I turned it off. The patient gasped and lapsed into unconsciousness again. I flicked it back on and her eyes popped open. When she asked what had happened I told her that a fuse had blown.

Cardiology interns were not allowed to see patients in the out-patients clinics. Wiser heads had learned that interns messing about with cardiac drugs on an out-patient basis was not a good idea as these drugs are very important and potentially dangerous. It was felt that junior doctors needed at least one year's experience before they could prescribe outside the cardiac unit. Any mistake could be rectified within the unit in a very short time but outside the unit the patients were on their own. While the senior members of the cardiac team were at the clinic, my partner Mary and I stayed in the unit and looked after the patients.

❖   ❖   ❖   ❖

During this time I had decided to apply for the GP rotation, a three-year course that included work in General Medicine, Casualty, Obstetrics and Gynaecology, and Paediatrics, followed by a year in General Practice training. There were only four places on the rotation and these were eagerly sought. I submitted my CV and was called for interview. One of the interviewing professors asked me which medical journals I read.

'None,' I said.

'And why is that, Doctor?' he asked, a little miffed.

'I work about ninety hours a week. I haven't time to read journals.'

The point was taken and a few days later I was thrilled to be told by the Professor of Medicine that I had been successful in my application.

On 1 July 1977 I registered as a full doctor and began my job as a senior house officer in the Mater Hospital. Switching hospitals was thought to give the new doctor or future GP wider experience and was seen as an advantage.

Legally I was now able to see patients in a private capacity. This was against hospital rules but what the hospital authorities didn't know couldn't hurt them – and I wasn't going to tell them.

Chapter 10

SHO in General Medicine

The team I was on during my first six months as a Senior House Officer (SHO) was the professorial team with two registrars, a senior and junior lecturer, myself as SHO in the middle and three honours interns. I was caught in the midst of a load of medical talent and felt suffocated. Everybody had to do their rounds every day but, oddly enough, the patients appeared to enjoy the enormous number of physical examinations.

As well as my rounds, I also had to be on duty. My first night on duty did not go to plan. Being new to the Mater Hospital, I did not know where the various wards were located. I had just got to bed when my cardiac arrest bleeper blasted me back to reality.

I snatched up the telephone. 'Where's the arrest?' I asked.

'St Patrick's ward,' said the operator.

St Patrick's ward could have been in Africa for all I knew. The operator told me roughly where the ward was and off I ran, pulling on my pants and shoes. I hadn't a clue where to go. I ran down one corridor, stopping at each door and breathlessly enquiring if they happened to have a cardiac arrest. I became a little hysterical when I pushed open a door and found myself in the car park. I wandered aimlessly around the hospital for about fifteen minutes before I finally found St Patrick's ward. The patient had been taken to the intensive care unit and I stood there feeling silly.

The next day I started on the top floor of the hospital and worked my way down to the basement, learning where various wards and departments were located. I never got lost again.

Joan and I got married halfway through this year and moved into our house when we returned from our honeymoon. Weekends on duty were particularly difficult as it meant leaving Joan on her own. Sometimes she came to medical parties with me. One such party was hosted by the coronary care unit in one of the other hospitals. During the evening two patients wandered into the party as the noise had kept them awake. When we were leaving, a white-coated figure was lurching down the corridor in front of us, mumbling away to himself and doing little dances.

'Who's that?' asked Joan.

'The casualty officer,' I explained.

We followed him into casualty, which thankfully was not as busy as usual. He climbed onto his desk and started to tap dance to entertain the patients. When he fell off, one of the registrars hauled him away and put him into bed. Some of the waiting patients were very disappointed.

Being on call meant admitting patients from casualty, an autonomous part of the hospital. Here the casualty officer reigned along with three other casualty officers who covered the whole twenty-four hours.

A patient would be seen by the casualty officer who would decide whether he or she needed to be admitted or not. The SHO would be called to offer further advice and the patient would finally be admitted by the interns. All human life came to casualty and here I felt at home. It was the closest thing to general practice in the hospital environment. It was where a junior doctor got to see things at first hand and had to decide the treatment. Patients' lives were in your hands. The only back-up was from the medical registrar on duty, but he or she was usually busy in another part of the hospital.

I had just finished admitting a patient with pneumonia one night when an ambulance came screaming in. The ambulance man rushed into casualty with a little bundle in his arms.

'It's a baby, Doc. Head injury. It looks bad.'

I took the baby from him and put it on a stretcher. A brief examination told me all I needed. The baby was breathing in short gasps, there was blood coming out of the left ear and one of the pupils was fixed and dilated.

'We need help,' I said to one of the nurses. 'Call an arrest.'

The bleepers went off around the hospital. The baby was chubby – a chubby ten-month-old boy – and this made it difficult to find a vein in his arm. The anaesthetist arrived and had the drip up and running in no time.

The registrar arrived and examined the baby. 'Phone neurosurgery in the Richmond Hospital and tell them to expect a baby in about five minutes,' said the on-call registrar, dismay etched on his face.

'His mother is in one of the other cubicles,' said the casualty officer. 'She wants to know what's going on.'

The baby was removed to the Richmond Hospital accompanied by one of the doctors. I went into the mother's cubicle, not knowing what to say. She had a large bruise on her forehead and her arm looked broken.

'What happened?' I asked as gently as possible.

'Will my baby be all right, Doctor?'

'He has a head injury. We have sent him to the Richmond Hospital for treatment.' I asked her again what had happened.

'We were hit straight on by a drunk. I was sitting in the front seat with the baby in my lap. When the other car hit me

I put my arm up to protect' – she started to cry – 'to protect myself. The baby's head was caught between the window and my forehead.'

When the neurosurgical registrar at the Richmond phoned us soon afterwards to tell us that the baby was dead, nobody was very surprised. The drunk who had caused the accident was also in a casualty bed. He was singing away, oblivious to the carnage he had caused. I wanted to kill him. I got the feeling no one would have stopped me if I had tried.

On duty the following week a casualty case arrived with a collapsed lung. He needed a chest drain to be inserted to reinflate the lung. I was called down.

'So, who's going to put the drain in?' I asked.

'You're the SHO, you put it in,' replied the casualty officer.

I had seen drains put in, I had never actually done the job. I called another doctor and told him our predicament.

'I don't know how to bung it in. Where's the surgical registrar?' he said.

'Up in the theatre with the aneurysm,' explained an intern.

The 'aneurism' had been rushed in, nearly unconscious. We had been trying to figure out what was wrong with him. We knew there was something wrong in his abdomen as it was swollen and tender and when we examined his stomach he moaned in pain. The x-rays were not very helpful and we were getting a little exasperated. Our problem was solved when he opened his eyes.

'Is it me aneurysm, Doctor?'

'Your what?' I asked in turn.

'Me aneurysm, has it leaked?'

Bingo! He had an aortic aneurysm, a blow-out of the body's main artery. The consultant was called in and off the patient went for surgery.

In the meantime we were dealing with the collapsed lung

and the chest drain. The other doctor looked at me. 'Come on up to the library.'

We spent fifteen minutes going through the procedure of how to insert a chest drain and returned to the patient who had not been appraised of our little problem. I prepared the patient's left chest wall, gave him a local anaesthetic and motioned to my colleague that all was ready. He made a small incision over the area with a scalpel and slipped the chest tube into the opening. A lot of push is needed to put in this type of tube and with an audible grunt he forced the instrument into the chest cavity. There was a whoosh of escaping air.

'Is he still alive?' he whispered. 'I didn't spike his heart, did I?'

The patient looked unconcerned. After all he was in the hands of experts.

Chapter 11
Casualty

Without a shadow of a doubt my six months as a casualty officer in the Mater Hospital was one of the most enjoyable times I had as a junior hospital doctor. I and the other casualty officers insisted that a locum casualty officer be employed to cover for us when we were off duty.

The locum casualty officer, Abdul, was from the Middle East, and he immersed himself in his work with great gusto, often making surprise appearances even when he was off duty. Late one night in casualty he told me that there was a patient with an incomprehensible accent up from the country looking for the ominous-sounding special clinic. These special clinics dealt daily with the clap, gonorrhoea, genital warts and 'a specific disease' – a euphemism for syphilis and other nasties that were the end result of bonking the wrong person at the wrong time.

I was sitting at my desk when Abdul brought over the farmer who seemed in no great hurry to have his problem tended to. He was very small person and stood very close to my desk

'What's the problem?' I asked.

'It's my dick, Doc,' he stammered out.

'Why don't you bring it to a watchmakers?'

It was his turn to be a little confused. 'I didn't know that watchmakers looked at dicks, Doc.'

It must have been the time of night. We were getting further and further away from each other. I thought perhaps he was a bit simple. He kept talking about his tick-tock. I put my hand gently on his leg and whispered.

'Bring it down to the local watchmaker. He'll have a look at it, clean it out, and put in a new spring if needed.'

We were both looking at each other closely. The staff nurse who was standing between us understood what was going on and was waiting expectantly to find out how far this would go.

The patient bent down and looked me straight in the eyes. 'Doc, it's my dick, my willy. There is something wrong with it.'

The light dawned. I sat back on the chair and pretended to yawn. 'I'm sorry but I am very tired. What you want is the special clinic which is closed. Perhaps I can help?'

I meant he should go over to a cubicle and drop his trousers. He dropped his trousers there and then, and slapped the problem member on the table. I took one look at it and leapt up from my chair. The locum backed away muttering what sounded like ancient Arabic curses.

'Keep that thing away from me!' I snapped a little too loudly. Everybody close by turned to look at the thing resting on my desk. One of the junior nurses gave a little squeak and hid behind the staff nurse.

I stared at the diseased member. It looked as if it had been run over by a tractor.

'How long has it been that way?' I asked mystified.

'About six weeks ago it started to look funny. My own doctor was a little bit cheesed off when he saw it. He told me to go to confession and tell the priest that I had been with a woman, and then he sent me up here.'

'Put it back in right now,' I ordered and I arranged for an

appointment with the VD specialist for the morning. 'In the meantime,' I continued, 'it would be advisable not to have a relationship with anybody.'

I wanted to add that he was not to have a relationship with any living thing, animal, human or vegetable. He pulled up his trousers and stood there for a few moments. The casualty was deathly quiet. No one could believe what they had seen.

It was obvious that the man still had something on his mind and I asked him what it was. He wanted to go down to one of the red light districts to look for a 'hoor'. I told him he wasn't to touch a 'hoor' – they might be frightened. He had certainly frightened me. When he had gone, I scrubbed my desk thoroughly to remove any traces of his willy. I thought it was quite likely to fall off before he got to the clinic the next morning.

❖   ❖   ❖   ❖

The desk I sat at was the 'casualty officer's desk'. In front of it were five chairs on which the non-urgent cases sat waiting to be seen by the doctor. There a patient sat while I was busy with the blood and guts of daily routine, the unconscious, the accidents, the bleeding, the patients drunk and on dope, the pneumonia, collapsed lungs (which I could now treat with no problem), the acute asthmatics and the dead.

On one occasion after a dreadfully busy night I sat behind my desk and called the first person over to sit beside me. He was fifteen years old and wore thick glasses. His father stood behind him. I was exhausted and just wanted to get the casualty cleared so that I could get a little rest. However this boy took the biscuit as regards complaints.

'What's the problem?' I asked.

He took a deep breath. 'I'm going blind,' he said in a loud

frightened voice.

I was concerned for the young man for blindness at his age was a tragedy. 'Why do you think you are going blind?' I asked.

'I'm playing with myself too much,' he cried.

I tried to keep a straight face and coughed hard to conceal my laughter.

'The priest told me I would go blind if I kept playing with it.'

Luckily his father was a very understanding man; he didn't complain to the hospital authorities when I laughed out loud. I reassured the boy that he wouldn't go blind and the fact that the strength of his glasses had recently been adjusted was merely coincidental.

Casualty was full of problems like this. An eighteen-year-old girl was brought in having had too much to drink. She had fallen down a flight of stairs and knocked herself out. As casualty officer I had the responsibility of looking after her. I counselled her on the unpleasant things that can happen to a lady when intoxicated and told her that she could leave in five minutes if she felt up to it.

As I walked back to my desk I noticed an old codger sitting beside it. He must have been about eighty years old. He was wearing a cap and was resting his head on his hands. He looked up at me and his eyes popped wide open. I thought he was going to collapse but he was staring over my shoulder at something behind me. I spun around and there before me was a Venus de Milo with arms. I gawked at her. The eighteen-year-old was totally naked.

'Doc, can I put my clothes on now?' she asked sweetly.

'Yes, yes, of course,' I stammered and turned to the bug-eyed old fellow.

'What can I do for you?'

He smiled at me and stood up. 'Nothing, Doc. Nothing at all. I've just been cured.' He winked at me and left swinging his cane without a care in the world.

❖　　❖　　❖　　❖

The staff nurse called me into a cubicle one afternoon to a healthy-looking man sitting on the stretcher with his boots on.

'What's the problem?' I asked.

'I've got a verruca on my head.'

'A verruca on your head?'

'Yeah, the Preparation H won't budge it.' I hadn't the heart to tell him that Preparation H is used for haemorrhoids. The 'verruca' turned out to be a papilloma. I removed it and as I put in some stitches he informed me that Preparation H was useless. 'I might as well have been shoving it up my arse.'

❖　　❖　　❖　　❖

The staff nurses in casualty appeared to be from a different stock than the hospital nurses, not better, just different. They would tell you what was wrong before you got to the patient. They would say things like: 'There's a bloke in No 4 with a chest pain and cough. It looks like pneumonia,' or 'Headache in No 6, I think she's been beaten up by the boyfriend.' But perhaps the best was: 'There's a fellow in No 6 who has a nasty dog bite on his testicles.'

'I beg your pardon,' I said to the staff nurse.

She brought me over to the unfortunate who had been walking up a Dublin street when for no obvious reason an Alsatian had taken a dislike to his testicles. As I examined the considerable damage, I could not disguise my feelings.

'Can you fix up me tackle, Doc?' the patient asked calmly.

His actual testicles appeared to be relatively uninjured with only one or two puncture wounds from the teeth. The scrotal skin was another matter.

'I think you should be admitted and have things fixed up. There shouldn't be any problem,' I said.

'I can't come into hospital, Doc. Can't you do it down here. I'm self-employed, family to look after, the works.' He looked worried.

I thought about it for a moment. I told him that I could fix him up but it might be a little uncomfortable. I cautioned him that the result might not be a hundred percent successful.

'Go ahead, Doc, sew me up,' issued forth bravely.

I gave whatever local anaesthetic I could and put the scrotum back into a shape that wouldn't frighten his wife. Each time I put in a stitch – there were thirty-eight altogether – I could feel tingles of sympathy in parts of my own body. When I had finished I stood back and appraised my work like an artist with an oil painting.

'What do you think?' I asked one of the nurses. She bent down close and inspected the work. It seemed to twitch a little.

'Looks fine,' she said hurriedly.

'Come back here in seven days and we'll take the stitches out,' I said.

The patient appeared satisfied with that and left casualty walking as if he had been in the saddle all day.

Suturing was one of the main jobs in casualty and my experience in America was invaluable. When I had the time I sutured anything that needed the job.

A Gaelic hurling player was brought in from Croke Park. He had a laceration that split his top lip, moved up the left side of his nose and into his forehead. I told him the options and again was told to go ahead. I used no local anaesthetic this time. Injecting local anaesthetic tends to distort the skin and when you are putting a face back together any distortion adds to the scar. He didn't flinch as I sutured him although it must have been exquisitely painful as the lips and the skin of the nose are very sensitive.

It was a quiet afternoon and I took my time. I put in about thirty stitches and when I had finished I knew the job was good.

When he returned two months later I was thrilled to see that there was practically no scar. It was one of the best suturing jobs I had ever done and I felt rightly proud of myself.

Unfortunately not all lacerations turn out so well. Drunks especially tend to move about while you attempt to repair the damage. On occasion they take a swing at you when you insert the needle!

Drunks were the curse of casualty. Saturday nights were 'fight nights' and a fight in casualty itself was common. If the police were not around we had no alternative but to let the fight continue until somebody was knocked out or they all fell down exhausted. Fights between women were especially fierce. The insults were novel and very personal. Clumps of hair flew about like little hairy UFOs, accompanied by screams and shouts. Inevitably the fight would reach a natural conclusion when one of the competitors would fall down and start to cry. Thankfully, injuries were never serious and after we had examined the combatants we would send them off to continue their altercation at some other address.

Drunks were seen to and then put into a room, commonly referred to as the 'drunk tank', with benches where they could sleep it off. One had to be very careful when a drunk was put in there. If they had a head laceration they would be checked every thirty minutes or so to make sure that they hadn't got a brain haemorrhage under the laceration. Every year I heard stories about casualty officers from many different hospitals who had failed to detect a brain haemorrhage and released the patient who, much to the casualty officer's embarrassment, would be brought back to casualty a few hours later, often dead.

I never missed a brain haemorrhage but I did miss broken hips, two of them, in the same patient. A mental patient from one of the outlying mental hospitals was found at the bottom of the stairs trying to stand up. The junior psychiatrist who phoned me about the case told me that the patient communicated by shouts, grunts and screams only. He had been examined but no major problem was found.

'But his grunts and screams are of a different pitch,' said the psychiatrist. 'We've never heard these ones before. We think he's broken something. Can we send him in to you?'

It sounded interesting. I could detect a challenge. When the patient arrived into casualty I examined him from head to foot. I asked the surgical registrar to examine him. I x-rayed his head, neck, chest, pelvis, both arms and hands. I think he received more internal damage from the x-rays than he had from his injuries. I phoned the psychiatrist, told him I had found nothing, and sent him back. A few hours later I had another look at his x-rays. They looked normal except for the pelvis. Something was wrong but for the love of me I couldn't see it. I wandered into the x-ray room.

'Did you see anything wrong with these hips?' I asked one of the two radiographers. Radiographers are not qualified doctors and strictly speaking are not meant to make diagnoses, but they knew more about x-rays than I did so it never bothered me to ask. They both had a look.

'Heads of both femurs have gone through the acetabula.' In other words, he had broken his pelvis on both sides. I grabbed the x-rays and held them close to the overhead light.

'Where?' I demanded, a little panic starting in my gut. They pointed out what I had failed to spot.

Cursing to myself I phoned the psychiatrist. 'Send him back,' I choked out.

'Why?'

'Femoral heads through the acetabula.' I swallowed hard. 'Both of them.'

'Oh, really? Well, well, well!'

I ate humble-pie. The patient was returned to us and transferred to the orthopaedic team on call.

❖   ❖   ❖   ❖

Out of the blue a case would present itself that defied explanation. One young man came in looking very worried and told me that he had been passing blood since early morning. Examination was normal as was his urine test, not a trace of blood found, although the sample he produced was bright red. He had no pains to indicate a stone in his kidney, his dangly bits were in good working order and he looked fine and healthy. I went through his history again and had a sudden flash of inspiration.

'You weren't by any chance eating beetroot last night?'

'I was actually,' he beamed. 'I ate half a jar of them.'

Somewhere in a dusty part of my brain a long dormant memory had flashed into my conscious with the information that too much beetroot turns urine red. Exit one very relieved young man.

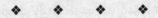

It was almost summer, time for me to apply for my job in Paediatrics. I was called for an interview in one of the children's hospitals. Being on the GP rotation didn't mean I was given the job automatically, but it would have come as a great surprise if I didn't get it. The interview went well and I was accepted as a junior hospital doctor for the six months from July. In the meantime I had to complete my casualty job.

As I was now an SHO, one of my duties was to teach the students, both medical and nursing, whatever I could. This completed the cycle – student/intern/teacher – except that I felt I didn't know that much more than the Final Med students. The only difference was that I had my degree. I showed them how to set up drips, suture, pass catheters and, most importantly, carry out cardiac resuscitation. From my days in St Vincent's I was confident of my ability to run a successful resuscitation. Whenever an arrest appeared the students didn't stand around and gawk. They were expected to help at the cardiac massage, setting up the drips and taking blood, on occasions they were allowed to defib the patient.

It was the same for anything that came through casualty. The students were allowed to examine patients and suggest treatments. They could suture any laceration under supervision, except faces and hands. To the best of my ability I allowed them what I had been allowed to do in America. Hands-on experience teaches more than theory in books. I tried to teach the junior nurses whenever the opportunity arose. Some were content to just do their 'ordinary jobs', others wanted 'to have a go'. Drunk patients with lacerations were the best to learn on, especially those with lacerations on their scalps. Here was a chance for the more adventurous nurse to learn how to suture. I would put in a few sutures and then hand over the instruments to the watching student nurse. I had to review my teaching technique when one of the young ladies sutured part of her glove into the wound with a dexterity that confounded me.

However, the patients and their relatives still never failed to amaze me. A young girl came in with an early urinary tract infection. I explained to her father that I was going to put her on an antibiotic after taking a test sample of urine and that I would send the result to her GP. He seemed happy with that but the next day he came back to inform me that he was reporting me to the Medical Board. Had his daughter died during the night? Had she developed some appalling reaction to the drug?

'The tablets are too cheap!' he bellowed.

'What?'

'The tablets are too cheap to work properly, I want more expensive ones.'

The drugs I had prescribed cost around two pounds. I wrote out a new prescription with humble apologies. I knew this new prescription would cost a small fortune. When the urine result came back, it showed the patient was sensitive to the cheap drug – that is the cheap drug worked – and resistant to the more expensive one. I immediately informed her GP and heard no more about it.

❖   ❖   ❖   ❖

My six months as a casualty officer ended on a down note. We lost a forty-six-year-old patient with asthma. He walked into casualty with his wife and within thirty minutes he was dead. No matter what we did we couldn't reverse his asthma. A whole team of doctors tried desperately to resuscitate him but it was no use. His wife, Martha, was in the waiting room expecting her husband to be treated and to go home.

'Tell her that things are not looking great,' I said to one of the staff nurses. I prepared Martha, just as Pat had shown me all those years ago in the States. Eventually the nurse brought Martha into the office where I gave her the bad news. I explained that we had lost the battle to save his life and that he had passed away.

'So, he won't be coming home tonight?' she said. Denial is something all doctors have to deal with. It is part of the grieving process and can last weeks or years.

'No, he won't be coming home tonight,' I said softly.

'I see, I see. When do you think he can come home?'

I took her by the shoulders and looked straight into her frightened eyes.

'He's dead, Martha. He won't be coming home at all. I am very sorry.'

'What will I tell the kids?' She started to cry. 'The youngest is only five years old. He's going to the carnival with him on Sunday.' She put her hand to her mouth. 'But he won't be going now, will he?'

I shook my head and whispered, 'I'm sorry.'

I felt my own eyes stinging. I had no more to say. I shuffled out of the room and leant against the wall. As Pat had said, you never get used to it.

Chapter 12

Paediatrics

𝓜y rotation in Paediatrics was divided into two months in Surgery, two months in Medicine and two months in the Paediatric Casualty. I was familiar with the hospital as I had been a student there with my friends from the reading room who were now scattered around the country. Surgery was fascinating. To watch the paediatric surgeon repairing a child was nothing short of miraculous but I wasn't able to do very much. The surgeons work in tiny spaces and there just isn't room for an extra pair of hands. The surgical SHO and registrar had to learn their craft and were present at all the operations. Even the neurosurgery which I still loved was a one-man job.

One of the consultants was somewhat intense and we didn't get on. There was a major personality clash that did not resolve itself even when I had left his team. He was a marvellous doctor and I would have no problem sending one of my children to him. However, I didn't enjoy my two months with that team.

One day I couldn't get a drip up on a pudgy baby. I had spent about twenty minutes trying to get the needle into a vein in the child's arm but to no avail. I had to call a consultant for help as both the registrar and SHO were busy. This consultant did not allow his team to put drips up in a child's scalp where it was very easy. He was not pleased to be called to do what was in reality a simple job.

'Can't put a drip up then, John?' he asked.

'Bet you five pounds you won't be able to find a vein,' I said stonily.

He accepted the bet and sat down by the bed. Some time later the drip was in place – in the child's scalp. I never collected my five pounds!

My worst moment in those two months of surgery was turning off the life support machine on a ten-year-old who had massive head injuries. In the morning, the neurosurgeon had examined the boy and decided to wait a few hours to see if there was any improvement in his condition. In fact we all knew it was hopeless, but hope springs eternal, especially when you are dealing with children. That afternoon the neurosurgeon phoned me and asked if there was any improvement. Sadly, the boy had not responded to any type of stimuli.

'Turn off the machine then. Can you deal with it?'

My heart sank. 'OK.'

His family were downstairs in the waiting-room, hoping for a miracle. I took a deep breath, wished him God speed and switched off the ventilator. Although he was hooked up to the ECG which recorded his heartbeat I sat on the chair beside the bed and put my stethoscope on his chest over his heart. I closed my eyes and waited for his death. I could feel the young body shift slightly when the oxygen was used up in his system. He seemed to stiffen a little as his heart gave one or two irregular beats and then stopped. I held my hand on his chest, lowered my head and sobbed.

The nurse came over to me and gently tapped me on the shoulder. 'It's over, John. You'd better tell the family. I'll fix things up here.'

Black despair was hanging over me. I freshened up in the toilet and went down the stairs to his waiting family. I stayed with them for about an hour. When I got home Joan knew I was in an emotional mess. We went out that night and I got very drunk.

❖   ❖   ❖   ❖

I breathed a sigh of relief when I joined one of the other teams for the two-month stint of my Paediatrics. It was a routine more attuned to general practice. I would start my ward rounds early in the morning and wait for the consultant to arrive. We would go over the charts and clinical problems of our new charges and finish around eleven.

We had a few cancer patients in the ward where I had dreaded to go as a student. Now it was different, I couldn't walk away as I had done before. I was part of the team and had to do my job. I tried to be as gentle as possible with these children and their courage made me feel very small indeed. They had tubes and drips poking into their bodies but they still managed to give me a smile even when I knew I was hurting them.

❖   ❖   ❖   ❖

I was also subjected to lots of abuse! In my first week as a paediatric casualty officer, I was spat at, vomited on, piddled and crapped on. I was threatened by worried parents and hit by a mother when I tried to suture her child. This was fairly normal and by the end of the first week I was used to the verbal abuse.

I was on duty one dark night when a man rushed in and told me that a child had fallen down a ditch and hurt his ankle. The child was out in the van and the man thought that his ankle was sprained. I wandered out and put my head into the van.

'What's the matter?' I asked the boy.

'Hurt me foot, Mister.' His foot was in the passenger well of the van and I couldn't see it. Prudently I ran my hand down his leg until I came to an unusual soggy lump. I asked for a torch and shone the beam at his ankle.

'Oh, shit!' I blurted out very unprofessionally. I backed out of the car and pointed. 'His bloody foot is hanging off!'

Very carefully I lifted him out of the car with his foot flapping around, hanging on by some tendons and ligaments. The ankle bones were totally exposed. The child was in shock and felt nothing. We wheeled him into the treatment room and set him down on the treatment table. There was surprisingly little bleeding. When the orthopaedic registrar arrived he stood in mute amazement at the end of the table. The consultant was called in and did the same thing. They spent most of the night in the operating theatre and I subsequently heard that the boy left the hospital a few weeks later with nothing more than a scar on his ankle.

I think I saved a tiny baby's life soon afterwards. A mother was walking past the hospital with her new baby boy in the pram. She looked down and saw that her baby had turned dark blue. With great presence of mind, she hauled him out of the pram and ran into casualty. She handed me the infant and just said, 'Please?'

There was no pulse, no breathing. I started doing cardiac massage immediately. I hadn't time to put up any drips, get any drugs, nothing. Just the cardiac massage and one breath into his lungs. Before the registrar arrived the baby was screaming to high heaven. The medical team took over and moved him to the intensive care unit. He was allowed home two days later, one of the few survivors of what appeared to be a near cot death.

But I experienced frustration and confrontation too. I had a few weeks in Paediatrics left when one morning a consultant arrived into my office with his team. We were very busy and his intrusion was not welcome. I stood up and asked what I could do for him. He told me that his SHO wanted to do a survey on the attendances at the casualty.

'That's very interesting. What has it got to do with me?' I asked.

'We want the casualty officers to fill out a questionnaire on every child they see. Each questionnaire will take only two to three minutes of your time.'

'Really? Only three minutes? I see about fifty to sixty kids a day. That means an extra two to three hours doing something that I haven't the time for.'

'I'm sure you'll find the time, Doctor,' he said stiffly.

'And if I decide to do this questionnaire will my name be at the top of the paper when it's published?'

'You'll be acknowledged at the end of the paper for your co-operation,' he replied.

'Hold on just a minute. I do the work, spend over two hours extra a day, on a paper that I don't want to do and I'll be "acknowledged" for my work?'

'That's right.'

I dug my heels in. 'I pass.'

'What!' he exclaimed.

'I pass. There is no way on earth that I'm going to do this survey. Get someone else who isn't busy to do it.'

'You have to do it,' he said.

I put my hands on the table and leaned towards him. 'No, I don't and if you'll excuse me, I have a bunch of kids outside, and I mean to see them.'

My heart was thumping. I had put my hands on the table to stop them shaking. The consultant stormed out of the room with his team in tow.

One of his juniors stopped at the door. 'You're crazy. You'll be fired,' he whispered.

'I don't give a shit!' I said, and I didn't.

❖   ❖   ❖   ❖

The paediatric casualty was always full. The holding ward, where we could put a child to bed to keep an eye on him or her, seldom had a free bed. There were a few cases that taught me more about families and children than many of the lectures I attended. I went into the holding area to examine a boy with a cough. His parents were sitting beside him and he didn't seem to be in great distress. The casualty was for urgent cases, not for 'kids with a cough', or KWACS as we called them. This KWAC was drinking some orange juice and appeared to be quite happy.

'Why didn't you bring him to your GP?' I asked his parents.

'We can't afford a doctor,' replied the mother.

I examined the child and sat on the bed. 'You should really bring him to his own GP in the morning,' I said. 'The casualty is no place for him.'

'We can't, we haven't got the medical card, Doctor. The money my husband earns is just over the limit to get a medical card. We'd be better off on the dole but he wants to work. Our money usually runs out before he gets paid. We don't drink or smoke and the money goes on food, rent, heat and electricity.'

I took a closer look at them and saw that their clothes were shabby, their shoes worn and holed and there were pieces of black twine instead of shoelaces. I had been brought up in a very comfortable middle-class environment – private school, holidays, pocket money – all these I had taken for granted. Poverty was something that happened to 'them'. Even as a casualty officer I had never really seen real poverty. I felt blinkered. I was about to give them a prescription for antibiotics when I saw the look in their eyes. They couldn't afford to get the medication for their child. I raided the drugs cupboard and gave them a week's supply and told them I would see what I could do about a medical card and any other benefits they might be entitled to. They thanked me and left.

When I saw the little boy a few days later he was very much improved. The parents had applied for an emergency medical card and on the strength of the letter that I had given them and a letter from one of the social workers, they had, against the odds, been granted one. At least the worry about medical expense was removed.

Another little lady taught me how children expressed stress and worry in childhood. She was brought in crying from a pain in her stomach. When I examined her she screeched out loud.

'Can you point to the spot that has the biggest hurt?' I asked her gently.

She pointed to her lefthand side, halfway between her pelvis and ribcage. The only organ of note in this area is the large bowel. Her parents had told me that she had done her 'poohs' and 'pees' quite normally that morning and had gone off to school. I wanted to examine her by herself and asked her parents to give me a few moments alone with her. When they left I knelt down beside the bed and put my hand on her stomach again. She made a face but didn't say anything. While I examined her, I asked her about her friends, her family, her pets and holidays. I left school until last. I told her about my pets and about the lioness named Flame that my mother used to look after.

She looked at me with big suspicious eyes. 'Your mum had a pet lion?'

'Well, not exactly a pet lion like a cat or a dog. But she used to go for walks with her in the zoo.'

'Really?' her big blue eyes shone with amazement.

I told her more stories, and made some up, about my mother who really *did* look after a lioness named Flame. After a while the pain seemed to go away. Then I asked her about school and I could feel her abdomen tighten again. Out of the blue she blurted out that one of her teachers didn't like her and she didn't want to go back to school. We talked for a few moments and I asked one of the nurses to bring her some orange juice. When she had finished I picked her up, put her on my back and carried her out to her anxious parents. I explained about the pain and school and suggested that they have a chat with the teacher who was an apparent worry to the child, real or imaginary. She skipped out of casualty holding her parents' hands.

❖   ❖   ❖   ❖

A child was brought in one day with a very nasty cough. I examined her and had her x-rayed. I also called down the medical registrar to have a look, just to make sure I didn't miss anything. I reassured her mother that everything was fine and decided that antibiotics were not indicated as it seemed to be a viral problem. I left for home that night happy in the knowledge that I appeared to have done a good day's work. When I came back the following morning I was stopped at the casualty door by the medical registrar. The child had been brought back in at about four o'clock in the morning very ill. She had severe pneumonia.

The parents were angry to say the least. The mother called me every name under the sun and even touched on my parentage. I re-examined the child and sure enough she had pneumonia. I went over my previous notes and looked at the x-rays we had done. They showed no sign of this infection. I decided that I had better talk to the parents but whatever I said was dismissed out of hand. As far as they were concerned I had let the child out with a serious illness and hadn't even put her on an antibiotic.

It was a no-win situation. I made my apologies humbly and left casualty as quickly as I could. It was one of the more unpleasant lessons I learned. When children get sick, they can get sick very quickly indeed. Explanations cut no ice with distraught parents. It's a lesson every doctor has to learn.

❖ ❖ ❖ ❖

It was now time to sit for the exam in child health. I was so busy in my private practice that I promised myself that if I didn't do as well as I had hoped I would repeat. Someday I'll have the time to do the repeat.

My time in Paediatrics was coming to a close but the kids did not stop coming to casualty. I removed small flowers from a kid's ears, peas from noses, tried to figure what 'technical colours in me eyes' meant and didn't once use words like penis, rectum or flatulence.

My private practice was in excellent shape but I still had another six months to do in Obstetrics and Gynaecology before I left hospital medicine for good.

Chapter 13

Obstetrics and Gynaecology

The National Maternity Hospital in Holles Street was one of the busiest maternity hospital in Europe, or so they told me. I was never allowed to forget that. Every student and junior hospital doctor was indoctrinated with this.

Some of the senior staff at the time had an unpleasant attitude towards the junior doctors. As far as they were concerned we knew nothing, although some of my colleagues had their membership in medicine, a degree not to be sniffed at. The ward sisters were the bosses and one of the chief bosses was in the delivery room. I had come across her as a lowly medical student and remembered her with some trepidation. Unfortunately, we started off on the wrong footing on my first weekend on duty. It was all about episiotomies.

Episiotomies are a surgical intervention in the birth of a baby, usually in a new mother about to give birth. The skin and tissue between the vagina and rectum can sometimes tear. A special surgical cut, called an episiotomy, can prevent a tear. After the birth of the baby the episiotomies have to be sewn up. Obviously, episiotomies can cause life-long problems if they are not properly looked after. Sex can be made very uncomfortable by the resultant scar tissue.

On my first night on call I was called to the delivery room

to sew up a new mum. Her episiotomy was very large. In my innocence I thought I could deal with it because of my short experience in plastic surgery, and that it would need a fair amount of sutures. I introduced myself to the patient, told her what I was going to do and settled myself down.

Repairing an episiotomy is not the most dignified operation for any woman, as a total stranger is sitting between her legs and putting needles in areas that really are not meant for them. Sometimes when I was in this unorthodox position I would flinch at the thought that if I hurt my patient her knees could smash my ears together. I began to repair the wound and got hopelessly lost. Plastic surgery and episiotomies, I began to realise, were miles apart. The old adage: if you don't know what to do, do nothing, came to mind and I hollered for help. The doctor on call came down, moved me out of the way and put in three big sutures. He stood up and left. That was the only tutoring I got in the art of repairing episiotomies.

The next case came in and again I had to do the repair. My training with Mr Murphy and Mr O Riain in plastic surgery again came to mind and I was beginning to see how I might apply the same approach in this situation. I started to repair the young lady to the best of my ability. Halfway through the procedure the staff sister came over to me.

'Aren't you finished yet?' she demanded.

'In about five minutes,' I answered.

'You've put in too many stitches there,' she said, peering at the nearly finished repair.

I could feel the hairs on the nape of my neck beginning to rise. A colleague, be it nurse or doctor, never ever, under any circumstances criticises the doctor in front of a patient. The patient's confidence is not helped by seeing her practitioner questioned on his technique.

'Let me ask you a question, Sister,' I whispered, loud enough for the patient to hear. 'Which would you prefer? My way,' and I pointed to the job I was just finishing 'or the other way?'

She looked me straight in the eyes. 'Well, hurry up. There is another waiting to be done,' she said and left.

❖   ❖   ❖   ❖

The out-patients department had not changed since I was there as a student but now as an SHO in gynaecology, I had my own patients to interview and treat, and used the consultant and assistant master to back me up if necessary. We always had students tagging along and were expected to teach them about various gynaecological cases. As they were going through their gynaecological rotation and swotting up for their exams they probably knew more about the subject at that time than I did. But sometimes I could teach them something new.

On one occasion a very pregnant woman appeared in my cubicle. She had been given an appointment by mistake and should have gone to the antenatal clinic.

'Do you mind if some students come in to examine you?' I asked her.

She shook her head. 'Not at all, I'm well used to it.'

Six students piled into the cubicle and stood around the bed. The patient was definitely used to students. She lifted her maternity smock and exposed her very big tummy and legs. The students were trying to look serious, doctor-like.

'Now, what is the very first thing you notice before examining the patient?' I asked. I could feel the dark side of myself gaining control.

'Well, she's very advanced in her pregnancy,' ventured one of the students.

'What else?' I asked.

'She has no stretch marks,' answered another, a little embarrassed by his answer.

'And what else?' I tempted.

The students looked at me and then at each other.

I sighed heavily. 'She's got a fabulous pair of legs.'

The patient burst out laughing. The students looked at me as if I had grown another head. The curtain was pulled back with a flourish and the consultant beckoned me out.

'You do *not* tell the patient that they have a fabulous pair of legs,' he said angrily.

'Why not? She's only pregnant and she has a fabulous pair of legs. She's laughing. What's wrong with that?'

'This is a hospital, not a comedy store.'

I had watched this consultant examining his patients before. He strolled into the cubicle without so much as an hello to the patient, examined them without looking at their faces and left. I apologised and returned to the students.

'Our patient here is only pregnant. She doesn't have a disease, she doesn't have a tumour. She is perfectly healthy and normal. With your permission,' I glanced at her and she nodded, 'we will examine her.'

They did her blood pressure, felt her abdomen, found the baby's head and listened with their stethoscopes.

'Hold on a second,' I said as they put away their stethoscopes, 'we've all heard the baby's heart, perhaps the patient would like to have a listen as well?'

I took my stethoscope from around my neck and gave it to the patient. She put the earpieces on and I put the bell of the stethoscope on to her abdomen. Her eyes lit up as she heard the fast heartbeat of her yet to be born baby. She listened for a few moments and handed the stethoscope back to me.

'Thank you, Doctor. I've never done that before.' She got up, pulled down her smock and left smiling.

❖　　❖　　❖　　❖

Every week I attended the infertility clinic with one of the consultants. I had always thought that 'getting pregnant' was easy and I didn't think it would be so very difficult for some couples. Some of the problems were insurmountable but occasionally the problems could be dealt with there and then. I was sitting with the consultant when a new patient presented herself. She had been trying to get pregnant for four years but with no luck. Her GP had sent her to the clinic without examining her or her husband. The consultant went through her gynaecological history. No problems there. Then he came to her sexual history.

'Any problems with sexual intercourse?' he asked.

She blushed a little. 'No, Doctor. No problems.'

'Good, good. Now how often would you have sexual intercourse?'

'On average about twice, Doctor.'

'I see, twice a week, twice a month?' he prompted.

'Twice a day,' she answered sweetly.

The consultant sat up straighter in his chair and cleared his throat. 'You have had sex twice a day, every day for the past four years?'

She nodded, 'Except during, you know, my monthlies. Is there something wrong with that?'

I wanted to see her husband. I wanted to examine him. I wanted to see what he weighed. The consultant shuffled in his chair.

'Is your husband with you today?' he enquired. He had to see this guy as well.

Her husband was outside in the waiting room and the consultant invited him in. I stood with the consultant and waited for the couple to appear. When they came back my initial reaction was correct – he weighed about eight stone. He was also about six feet tall and to say that he was thin was an exaggeration. He was gaunt. He looked anorexic. We introduced ourselves, barely able to restrain the awe we felt for this matchstick. We went through their sexual history once again, just to make sure we had heard it correctly. The consultant explained about sperm count and infertility. The man needed to do a test called a Huhner's test to measure the amount of sperm he produced. The consultant asked them to refrain from sex for two weeks before the husband produced his sample.

'His sample of what?' asked the wife.

'A sperm sample,' the consultant replied.

'How will I get that?' the man asked.

'Well, the best way is by masturbation and the sample is collected into a little container we'll give you.'

'You mean you have to,' he gulped, 'I have to whack myself?'

'Well, there's another way, but masturbation is the best. Do you have any problems with this?'

'You mean we shouldn't make love for two weeks and then I have to . . .' he hesitated, 'and then I have to produce the goods?' He smiled and looked at his wife. He looked relieved at the prospect of two weeks' rest. His wife looked thoughtful. Perhaps she was relieved as well. A well-earned holiday for them.

Two weeks later the sample was produced. He was a very healthy young man. The couple were advised to abstain for two weeks until his wife was in the middle of her menstrual cycle. Eight weeks later she presented herself at the antenatal clinic six weeks pregnant.

Not all cases were as easy as this. My heart would break when couples were told they had little chance of conceiving. Joan was twelve weeks into her first pregnancy and all seemed to be going well. The thought of not having a family never once entered my mind. This arrogance was going to get one hell of a blow in the following weeks.

As a gynaecological SHO I had to deal with the miscarriages that presented at Holles Street. The patients came in, were diagnosed, had a small operation to clear out what remained and were usually sent home the next day. Unfortunately, I took a somewhat cavalier attitude to these problems at the beginning. I never thought that these women had lost a baby, merely that they had expelled a collection of cells and tissue that had failed to become a baby, a 'blighted ovum'. I couldn't get as upset as they were. Until my wife had a miscarriage. Thankfully I was on holiday and working at home on my private practice. I was showing a patient out when Joan called me upstairs.

'I'm bleeding, John,' she said softly. I reassured her as best I could and put her to bed, hoping that the bleeding would stop in the next twenty-four hours. It didn't and I decided she needed a scan. We went to the hospital where she was admitted to the unit where I was SHO. We went down to the scan room and I waited, full of dread. The signs were not good and the radiographer shook her head gently. Joan was having a miscarriage. The evacuation operation was soon over and when I went back in to see Joan, she was wide awake. I couldn't look into her eyes.

'Hi,' she said brightly.

I was a little confused. I felt worse than she did.

But the next morning we were both hit with the emotional loss. Joan described her sense of loss, the empty feeling she had, the feeling that something was wrong with her, that perhaps she couldn't have a baby. I had never considered these questions when a woman came in with a miscarriage. But the nail that sealed the coffin as regards my macho ideas came a few weeks later when I was examining a woman who was bleeding. She miscarried into my gloved hands. I saw what she didn't. A tiny twelve-week-old foetus in the palm of my hand. I closed my hand over the little body and put it into a kidney tray. I reassured the lady that all was well and that she had had a 'blighted ovum', that there would be no effect whatsoever on her next pregnancy.

Doing hysterectomies on patients who were well advanced in their pregnancies for cancer made me think about 'therapeutic abortions' more and more. I finally came to the conclusion that for reasons other than to save the life of the mother abortions were wrong. I have had patients who felt that an abortion was the only way for them and I have helped them to the best of my ability, and made sure that they came back to me after their trip to England. I have never judged one of these ladies and never will.

❖　　❖　　❖　　❖

Crises of different types could crop up and catch me unprepared. I was interviewing a lady who had a prolapsed womb that needed repair, possibly a hysterectomy. She had five children and I asked her to discuss the problem with her husband. She looked at me blankly.

'Me what?'

'Your husband,' I said.

'My husband fecked off after the second baby was born,' she informed me.

'What about the other three babies?' I asked cautiously.

'The first was a night of passion and love with a stranger, and the last two were with my boyfriend.'

I explained that it would be best if she used some form of contraception, French letters perhaps, until we got things sorted out.

'Frenchies! They're against the Church!' she nearly shouted. 'I won't let him near me until after the operation, you can be sure of that. If you do a repair, can you do a tubal litigation as well?'

I was knocked off balance again. 'A tubal litigation? I think you mean a tubal ligation, tying off the Fallopian tubes.'

She nodded her head vigorously. 'Yeah, that's right. Tie me tubes.'

In those days, as a Catholic hospital, the National Maternity Hospital had a very strict ban on tubal ligations. I heard that in some hospitals one would occasionally be sneaked in when a Caesarian section was performed and it had been requested by the patient. It is only fairly recently that this ban has been thrown out. I discussed the case with the consultant, and he suggested a hysterectomy.

'Will you suck it out of me with a Hoover?'

'Yes,' I said with complete understanding. 'We will suck it out with a Hoover. You will have no scar, nothing.' I was learning how to translate!

She seemed happy with the added bonus of no more pregnancies and accepted our offer of a vaginal hysterectomy.

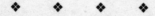

It was traditional that the SHO in gynaecology arranged the patients for the Final Medical examination. I was asked to be the official invigilator for that year's exams. The night before the exams I went around the wards asking patients if they would mind being a subject for the students. Without exception they gave their permission to be prodded and poked by inexperienced hands. There were six obstetrics, three postnatal, three antenatal and six gynaecological cases.

The students were waiting in the same library that I had sat in with such trepidation a few years before. I had had a few breaks in my student days with the exams. Perhaps I could repay the debt now, I thought. I went into the library and looked at the nervous faces.

'Who wants gynae cases and who wants obstetrics cases?' I asked calmly. Their mouths opened in unison. I pointed to a girl in the front row and asked her. 'What would you like? Obs or Gobs.'

'Obs, please.'

'Antenatal or postnatal?'

'Antenatal, please.'

They all got what they wanted. They all passed their exams. It's nice to have a break now and again.

❖   ❖   ❖   ❖

My own private practice was now well under way and my dad was under pressure when I was at the hospital. The hospital authorities obviously didn't know about my outside job – it was against the rules to run a practice outside the hospital.

In the middle of the out-patients clinic a senior consultant told me that he had a patient who needed a GP in my area and would I be so kind as to take her on.

'Sure,' I said and that was that. I was never cautioned or told that I was breaking the rules of my contract. My own private practice didn't interfere with my hospital job and I made sure that the hospital job didn't interfere with my private practice.

The rotation I was now in demanded that I spend a year in another practice as a trainee GP. This would have meant economic suicide. I told the GP co-ordinator that I could not leave my own practice but he was adamant. I tried to explain that as far as GP trainers were concerned my father had practically written the book on how to become a GP.

The GP co-ordinator said he understood my problem and hinted that if I didn't do what was required I might be expelled from the scheme.

I had had enough of medical politics and that night after a particularly busy surgery and heavy heart I resigned from the GP training scheme.

I was the last doctor in my six-month rotation group on duty and on the the first of July I finished night duty, ran down the stairs of the hospital, whipped off my white coat and gave a V-sign to hospital medicine and entered private practice full time.

I am still here. There will be no more stories.

Other Books from The O'Brien Press

PERSONAL HEALTH RECORD

A passport-sized permanent record for all information about your family's health from birth onwards. Invaluable.

£3.99 hb

A THORN IN THE SIDE
Fr Pat Buckley

The story of his life and career, and thoughts on issues of contemporary life, from this radical priest.

£9.99 pb

UNIVERSITIES & COLLEGES IN THE UK
The Irish Student's Essential Guide
P.M. McGoldrick

The best guide for all students thinking of third-level study in the UK. Fully comprehensive.

£7.99 pb

THE OUTRAGEOUS GUIDE TO THE WORLD CUP
Paul Farrell & Graeme Keyes

An outrageously funny and irreverent guide to the World Cup – its history, the teams, the countries, the grandparent rule; Irish football from St Patrick to Jack Charlton. Lots of cartoons.

£4.99 pb

THE OFFICIAL GREEN ARMY JOKE BOOK
John Byrne

80 pages chockful of jokes and cartoons about football, the players, the journalists, the fans, the Boss. The essential pocket-size, take-anywhere accessory for fans aged nine to ninety.

£3.50 pb

LOTTERY
Michael Scott

Winning the Lottery catapults Christine Quinn into the world
of the super-rich. Then dark shadows of her nightmare past
appear, threatening to destroy her new-found happiness.

£4.99 pb

A VOICE FOR SOMALIA
President Mary Robinson

A first-hand account by the President of her historic visit to
famine-stricken Somalia; her day-by-day diary, and hopes and
suggestions for the future.

£6.95 pb

A BOOK OF IRISH QUOTATIONS
Edited by Sean McMahon

'A major insight into Ireland...' J.P. Donleavy, IRISH LITERARY
REVIEW

£5.95 hb

ORDER FORM

Please send me the books as marked
I enclose cheque / postal order for £......... (+ 50p P&P per title) OR please
charge my credit card

☐ Access / Mastercard ☐ Visa

CARD NUMBER ☐☐☐☐ ☐☐☐☐ ☐☐☐☐ ☐☐☐☐
EXPIRY DATE ☐ ☐ ☐☐

NAME:...TEL:...
ADDRESS:...
....

Please send orders to : THE O'BRIEN PRESS, 20 VICTORIA ROAD, DUBLIN 6.
Tel: (Dublin) 4923333 Fax: (Dublin) 4922777